Innovation and Change in Professional Education

Volume 15

Series editor

Wim H. Gijselaers, School of Business and Economics, Maastricht University,
The Netherlands

Associate editors

L.A. Wilkerson, Dell Medical School at the University of Texas at Austin, TX, USA
H.P.A. Boshuizen, Center for Learning Sciences and Technologies,
Open Universiteit Nederland, Heerlen, The Netherlands

Editorial Board

Eugene L. Anderson, Anderson Policy Consulting & APLU, Washington, DC, USA
Hans Gruber, Institute of Educational Science, University of Regensburg,
Regensburg, Germany
Rick Milter, Carey Business School, Johns Hopkins University, Baltimore, MD, USA
Eun Mi Park, JH Swami Institute for International Medical Education,
Johns Hopkins University School of Medicine, Baltimore, MD, USA

SCOPE OF THE SERIES

The primary aim of this book series is to provide a platform for exchanging experiences and knowledge about educational innovation and change in professional education and post-secondary education (engineering, law, medicine, management, health sciences, etc.). The series provides an opportunity to publish reviews, issues of general significance to theory development and research in professional education, and critical analysis of professional practice to the enhancement of educational innovation in the professions.
The series promotes publications that deal with pedagogical issues that arise in the context of innovation and change of professional education. It publishes work from leading practitioners in the field, and cutting edge researchers. Each volume is dedicated to a specific theme in professional education, providing a convenient resource of publications dedicated to further development of professional education.

More information about this series at http://www.springer.com/series/6087

Olle ten Cate • Eugène J.F.M. Custers
Steven J. Durning
Editors

Principles and Practice of Case-based Clinical Reasoning Education

A Method for Preclinical Students

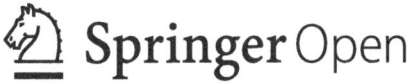

Editors
Olle ten Cate
Center for Research and Development
of Education
University Medical Center Utrecht
Utrecht, The Netherlands

Eugène J.F.M. Custers
Center for Research and Development
of Education
University Medical Center Utrecht
Utrecht, The Netherlands

Steven J. Durning
Uniformed Services University of the
Health Sciences
Bethesda, MD, USA

ISSN 1572-1957   ISSN 2542-9957   (electronic)
Innovation and Change in Professional Education
ISBN 978-3-319-87882-9   ISBN 978-3-319-64828-6   (eBook)
https://doi.org/10.1007/978-3-319-64828-6

© The Editor(s) (if applicable) and The Author(s) 2018. This book is an open access publication.
Softcover reprint of the hardcover 1st edition 2017
Open Access This book is licensed under the terms of the Creative Commons Attribution 4.0 International License (http://creativecommons.org/licenses/by/4.0/), which permits use, sharing, adaptation, distribution and reproduction in any medium or format, as long as you give appropriate credit to the original author(s) and the source, provide a link to the Creative Commons license and indicate if changes were made.
The images or other third party material in this book are included in the book's Creative Commons license, unless indicated otherwise in a credit line to the material. If material is not included in the book's Creative Commons license and your intended use is not permitted by statutory regulation or exceeds the permitted use, you will need to obtain permission directly from the copyright holder.
The use of general descriptive names, registered names, trademarks, service marks, etc. in this publication does not imply, even in the absence of a specific statement, that such names are exempt from the relevant protective laws and regulations and therefore free for general use.
The publisher, the authors and the editors are safe to assume that the advice and information in this book are believed to be true and accurate at the date of publication. Neither the publisher nor the authors or the editors give a warranty, express or implied, with respect to the material contained herein or for any errors or omissions that may have been made. The publisher remains neutral with regard to jurisdictional claims in published maps and institutional affiliations.

Printed on acid-free paper

This Springer imprint is published by Springer Nature
The registered company is Springer International Publishing AG
The registered company address is: Gewerbestrasse 11, 6330 Cham, Switzerland

Preface

Probably the most core characteristic of any physician is their clinical reasoning ability as it touches all aspects of patient care. While this statement is not disputed, the education to support students in acquiring this ability is far from clear. Clinical reasoning has been the subject of substantial research to (1) clarify what it actually is; (2) identify when and why clinical reasoning goes wrong, resulting in errors or suboptimal care; (3) identify teaching approaches; and (4) recognize models of assessment. While some medical education scholars question whether clinical reasoning can be explicitly taught at all, the literature provides many teaching methods. None of these are conclusive and every medical school has their own way to support medical students in their development of clinical reasoning ability.

One area where there is agreement in the medical education community, based on a body of empirical work, is that clinical experience and a substantial knowledge base are necessary to reach high levels of clinical reasoning ability. Schools desiring to optimally *prepare* students for their clinical experiences face a difficult problem. How to best train students to think like a doctor? Can they learn taking histories and conducting physical examinations, formulating differential diagnoses, and proposing management plans *before* they enter the clinical arena? Integrated curricula, particularly in a vertical sense, attempt to combine basic science teaching with patient-based clinical teaching at early stages of the medical curriculum to optimize this preparation. But what if clinical experience itself is necessary to begin acquiring clinical reasoning ability?

This book describes a teaching method that has been used for over 20 years and has survived multiple medical curricula in different educational institutions in the Netherlands and other countries. The method is derived from the primary editor's Ph.D. studies on peer teaching in the 1980s at the University of Amsterdam Medical School.

In the past 10 years, the model has been used to support the modernization of medical curricula through EU-funded projects in Moldova, Georgia, Azerbaijan, and Ukraine. The most recent of these projects (MUMEENA or Modernizing Undergraduate Medical Education in the Eastern Neighboring Area) has led to a detailed, extensive description of the case-based clinical reasoning (CBCR) method that was first published as a gray-literature English language book and subsequently translated in the Georgian, Azeri, Ukrainian, and Spanish languages.

This volume was fully revised and expanded, resulting in the current publication.

The CBCR educational method is one approach to preparing students to think like doctors before they become engaged in patient care. We do not claim that it is the only (or even the preferred) method. What we can say is that this method has served many generations (thousands of medical students) in their preclinical period. Available student evaluations have been consistently as good as or better than other preclinical courses. The method can be applied within or added to an existing medical curriculum, as a core, elective, or extracurricular course.

The book has three parts. For readers interested in general understanding of clinical reasoning education, Part I (Chaps. 1, 2, 3, 4, and 5) will provide food for thought. For those interested to apply the CBCR method, Part II (Chaps. 6, 7, 8, 9, and 10) is recommended. Part III (the appendices) provides cases that can be used, for instance, by educators who wish to try out this method with their learners.

We wish to thank the many individuals who have contributed to the success of the CBCR method by being involved in the initial design, notably Professor Bert Schadé from the Academic Medical Center in Amsterdam, or by serving as consultants and by writing cases. For this volume, we thank Drs. Charles Magee, Mary Kwok, Jeremy Perkins, and Lieke van Imhoff for writing or editing one or more cases included in the appendix.

Utrecht, The Netherlands	Olle ten Cate
Utrecht, The Netherlands	Eugène J.F.M. Custers
Bethesda, MD, USA	Steven J. Durning

Contents

Part I Backgrounds of Educating Preclinical Students in Clinical Reasoning

1 Introduction.. 3
   Olle ten Cate

2 Training Clinical Reasoning: Historical
   and Theoretical Background.................................. 21
   Eugène J.F.M. Custers

3 Understanding Clinical Reasoning from Multiple Perspectives:
   A Conceptual and Theoretical Overview........................ 35
   Olle ten Cate and Steven J. Durning

4 Prerequisites for Learning Clinical Reasoning................. 47
   Judith L. Bowen and Olle ten Cate

5 Approaches to Assessing the Clinical Reasoning
   of Preclinical Students....................................... 65
   Olle ten Cate and Steven J. Durning

Part II The Method of Case-Based Clinical Reasoning Education

6 Case-Based Clinical Reasoning in Practice..................... 75
   Angela van Zijl, Maria van Loon, and Olle ten Cate

7 Assessment of Clinical Reasoning Using the CBCR Test.......... 85
   Olle ten Cate

8 Writing CBCR Cases.. 95
   Olle ten Cate and Maria van Loon

9	**Curriculum, Course, and Faculty Development for Case-Based Clinical Reasoning** .... Olle ten Cate and Gaiane Simonia	109
10	**A Model Study Guide for Case-Based Clinical Reasoning** .... Maria van Loon, Sjoukje van den Broek, and Olle ten Cate	121

Appendix 133

Index 205

Editors and Contributors

About the Editors

Olle ten Cate, Ph.D. is a professor of medical education and director of the Center for Research and Development of Education at University Medical Center Utrecht, The Netherlands. He was the originator and has been intermittently coordinator of CBRC courses from 1993 until 1999 in Amsterdam and from 2005 until 2016 in Utrecht. His research and development interests include curriculum development, peer teaching, competency-based medical education, clinical reasoning, and many other areas.

Eugène J.F.M. Custers, Ph.D. is a researcher in medical education at the Center for Research and Development of Education at University Medical Center Utrecht, The Netherlands. His primary area of expertise is clinical reasoning, the role of basic sciences in medical expertise, and illness script development. He also has a special interest in the history of medical education.

Steven J. Durning, M.D., Ph.D. is professor of medicine and pathology and director for the graduate programs in health professions education, the Introduction to Clinical Reasoning medical school course, and the Long-Term Career Outcome Study at the Uniformed Services University of the Health Sciences, Bethesda, Maryland, USA. He holds a Ph.D. in health professions education and is a practicing internist. His research and development interests include clinical reasoning, assessment, educational theory, peer teaching, and several other areas.

About the Contributors

Judith L. Bowen, M.D. is professor of medicine in the Division of General Internal Medicine and Geriatrics, Oregon Health and Science University, Portland, Oregon, USA, where she directs the Education Scholars Program, a longitudinal faculty development program for clinical teachers. She is a Ph.D. candidate in medical education at Utrecht University. Her research interests include clinical reasoning and curriculum with a focus on the impact of transitions of clinical responsibility on learning diagnostic reasoning.

Gaiane Simonia, M.D., Ph.D. is professor of internal medicine, head of the Division of Geriatrics, and head of the Department of Medical Education, Research and Strategic Development at Tbilisi State Medical University, Tbilisi, Georgia. She was involved as primary initiator of the MUMEENA project of modernizing medical education in Eastern European countries which included the introduction of CBCR in curricula in Georgia, Azerbaijan, and Ukraine.

Sjoukje van den Broek, M.D. is an assistant professor at the Unit of Medical Education, with an adjunct attachment with the Center for Research and Development of Education, both at University Medical Center Utrecht, The Netherlands. She has been involved with CBCR from 2010 as consultant and is currently a coordinator of the CBCR course for second-year medical students. She is also a Ph.D. candidate in medical education, and she supports, as general secretary, the Ethical Review Board for Health Professions Education Research of The Netherlands Association for Medical Education.

Maria van Loon, M.D. worked as a junior teacher at the Center for Research and Development of Education, University Medical Center Utrecht, The Netherlands. She was involved with CBCR in 2014 as a consultant and as a coordinator of the CBCR course for second-year medical students and was actively involved with the training of medical schools with CBCR in Georgia, Azerbaijan, Ukraine, and Spain. She now works as a resident in general practice at University Medical Center Utrecht.

Angela van Zijl, M.D. worked as a junior teacher at the Center for Research and Development of Education, University Medical Center Utrecht. She was involved with CBCR in 2013 as a coordinator of the CBCR course for second-year medical students and was actively involved with the training of medical schools with CBCR in Azerbaijan. At the moment, she is a resident in pediatrics at Gelderse Vallei Hospital Ede, The Netherlands.

Part I
Backgrounds of Educating Preclinical Students in Clinical Reasoning

Chapter 1
Introduction

Olle ten Cate

Clinical reasoning is a professional skill that experts agree is difficult and takes time to acquire, and, once you have the skill, it is difficult to explain what you actually do when you apply it—clinical reasoning then sometimes even feels as an easy process. The input, a clinical problem or a presenting patient, and the outcome, a diagnosis and/or a plan for action, are pretty clear, but what happens in the doctor's mind in the meantime is quite obscure. It can be a very short process, happening in seconds, but it can also take days or months. It can require deliberate, painstaking thinking, consultation of written sources, and colleague opinions, or it may just seem to happen effortless. And "reasoning" is such a nicely sounding word that doctors would agree captures what they do, but is it always reasoning? Reasoning sounds like building a chain of thoughts, with causes and consequences, while doctors sometimes jump at a conclusion, sometimes before they even realize they are clinically reasoning. Is that medical magic? No, it's not. Laypeople do the same. Any adult witnessing a motorcycle accident and seeing a victim on the street showing a lower limb in a strange angle will instantly "reason" the diagnosis is a fracture. Other medical conditions are less obvious and require deep thinking or investigations or literature study. Whatever presentation, doctors need to have the requisite skills to tackle the medical problems of patients that are entrusted to their care. No matter how obscure clinical reasoning is, students need to acquire that ability. So how does a student begin to learn clinical reasoning? How must teachers organize the training of students?

Case-based clinical reasoning (CBCR) education is a design of training of preclinical medical students, in small groups, in the art of coping with clinical problems as they are encountered in practice. As will be apparent from the description

O. ten Cate (✉)
Center for Research and Development of Education, University Medical Center Utrecht,
Utrecht, The Netherlands
e-mail: T.J.tenCate@umcutrecht.nl

© The Author(s) 2018
O. ten Cate et al. (eds.), *Principles and Practice of Case-based Clinical Reasoning Education*, Innovation and Change in Professional Education 15,
https://doi.org/10.1007/978-3-319-64828-6_1

later in this chapter, CBCR is not identical to problem-based learning (Barrows and Tamblyn 1980), although some features (small groups, no traditional teacher role) show resemblance. While PBL is intended as a method to arrive at personal educational objectives and subsequently acquire new knowledge (Schmidt 1983), CBCR has a focus on training in the application of systematically acquired prior knowledge, but now in a clinical manner. It aims at building illness scripts—mental representations of diseases—while at the same time supports the acquisition of a diagnostic thinking habit. CBCR is not an algorithm or a heuristic to be used in clinical practice to efficiently solve a new medical problem. CBCR is no more and no less than *educational method* to acquire clinical reasoning skill. That is what this book is about.

The elaboration of the method (Part II and III of the book) is preceded in Part I by chapters on the general background of clinical reasoning and its teaching.

What Is Clinical Reasoning?

Clinical reasoning is usually defined in a very general sense as "The thinking and decision -making processes associated with clinical practice" (Higgs and Jones 2000) or simply "diagnostic problem solving" (Elstein 1995).

For the purpose of this book, we define clinical reasoning as the mental process that happens when a doctor encounters a patient and is expected to draw a conclusion about (a) the nature and possible causes of complaints or abnormal conditions of the patient, (b) a likely diagnosis, and (c) patient management actions to be taken. Clinical reasoning is targeted at making decisions on gathering diagnostic information and recommending or initiating treatment. The mental reasoning process is interrupted to collect information and resumed when this information has arrived.

It is well established that clinicians have a range of mental approaches to apply. Somewhat simplified, they are categorized in two thinking systems, sometimes subsumed under the name *dual-process theory* (Eva 2005; Kassirer 2010; Croskerry 2009; Pelaccia et al. 2011). Based in the work of Croskerry (2009) and the Institute of Medicine (Balogh et al. 2015), Fig. 1.1 shows a model of how clinical reasoning and the use of System 1 and 2 thinking can be conceptualized graphically.

The first thinking approach is rapid and requires little mental effort. This mode has been called *System 1 thinking* or *pattern recognition*, sometimes referred to as non-analytical thinking. Pattern recognition happens in various domains of expertise. Based on studies in chess, it is estimated that grand master players have over 50,000 patterns available in their memory, from games played and games studied (Kahneman and Klein 2009). These mental patterns allow for the rapid comparison of a pattern in a current game with patterns stored in memory and for a quick decision which move to make next. This huge mental library of patterns may be compared with the mental repository of *illness scripts* that an experienced clinician has and that allows for the rapid recognition of a pattern of signs and symptoms in a

1 Introduction

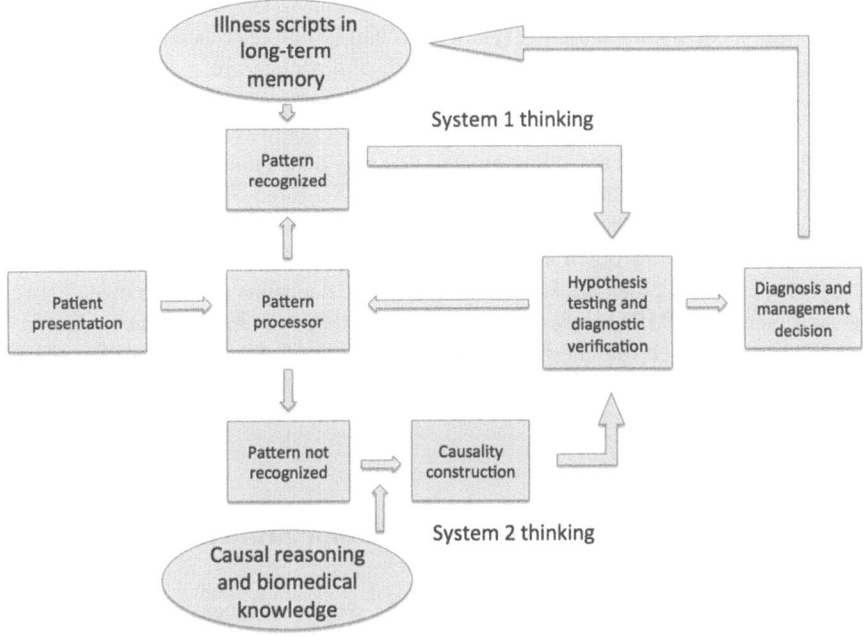

Fig. 1.1 A model of clinical reasoning (Adapted from Croskerry 2009)

> **Box 1.1 Illness Script**
> An illness script is a general representation in the physician's mind of an illness. An illness script includes details on typical causal or associated preceding features ("enabling conditions"); the actual pathology ("fault"); the resulting signs, symptoms, and expected diagnostic findings ("consequences"); and, added to the original illness script definition (Feltovich and Barrows 1984), the most likely course and prognosis with suitable management options ("management"). An illness script may be stored as one comprehensive unit in the long-term memory of the physician. It can be triggered to be retrieved during new clinical encounters, to facilitate comparison and contrast, in order to generate a diagnostic hypothesis.

patient with patients encountered in the past (Feltovich and Barrows 1984; Custers et al. 1998). See Box 1.1.

A mental matching process can lead to an instant recognition and generation of a hypothesis, if sufficient features of the current patient resemble features of a stored illness script.

Next to this rapid mental process, clinicians use *System 2 thinking:* the *analytical thinking mode of presumed causes-and-effects reasoning* that is slow and takes effort and is used when a System 1 process does not lead to an acceptable proposition to act. Analytic, often pathophysiological, thinking is typically the approach that textbooks of medicine use to explain signs and symptoms related to pathophysiological conditions in the human body. Both approaches are needed in clinical health care, to arrive at decisions and actions and to retrospectively justify actions taken. The two thinking modes can be viewed on a cognitive continuum between instant recognition and a reasoning process that may take a long time (Kassirer et al. 2010; Custers 2013). In routine medical practice, the rapid *System 1* thinking prevails. This thinking often leads to correct decisions but is not infallible. However, the admonition to slow down the thinking when System 1 thinking fails and move to System 2 thinking may not lead to more accurate decisions (Norman et al. 2014). In fact, emerging fMRI studies seem to indicate that in complex cases, inexperienced learners search for rule-based reasoning solutions (System 2), while experienced clinicians keep searching for cases from memory (System 1) (Hruska et al. 2015).

How to Teach Clinical Reasoning to Junior Students?

It is not exactly clear how medical students acquire clinical reasoning skills (Boshuizen and Schmidt 2000), but they eventually do, whether they had a targeted training in their curriculum or not. Williams et al. found a large difference in reasoning skill between years of clinical experience and across different schools (Williams et al. 2011). Even if reasoning skill would develop naturally across the years of medical training, it does not mean that educational programs cannot improve.

One way to approach the training of students in clinical reasoning is to focus on things that can go wrong in the practice of clinical reasoning and on threats to effective

---

Box 1.2 Summary of Prevalent Causes of Errors and Cognitive Biases
Errors (Graber et al. 2005; Kassirer et al. 2010)

- Lack or faulty knowledge
- Omission of, or faulty, data gathering and processing
- Faulty estimation of disease prevalence
- Faulty test result interpretation
- Lack of diagnostic verification

Biases (Balogh et al. 2015)

- Anchoring bias and premature closure (stop search after early explanation)
- Affective bias (emotion-based deviance from rational judgment)
- Availability bias (dominant recall of recent or common cases)
- Context bias (contextual factors that mislead)

thinking in clinical care. Box 1.2 shows the most prevalent errors and cognitive biases in clinical reasoning (Graber et al. 2005; Kassirer et al. 2010). See also Chap. 3.

In general, diagnostic errors are considered to occur too often in practice (McGlynn et al. 2015; Balogh et al. 2015), and it is important that student preparation for clinical encounters be improved (Lee et al. 2010). In a qualitative study, Audétat et al. observed five prototypical clinical reasoning difficulties among residents: generating hypotheses to guide data gathering, premature closure, prioritizing problems, painting an overall picture of the clinical situation, and elaborating a management plan (Audétat et al. 2013), not unlike the prevalent errors in clinical practice as summarized in Box 1.2. Errors in clinical reasoning pertain to both System 1 and System 2 thinking and cognitive biases causing errors are not easily amenable to teaching strategies. An inadequate knowledge base appears the most consistent reason for error (Norman et al. 2017). A number of authors have recommended tailored teaching strategies for clinical reasoning (Rencic 2011; Guerrasio and Aagaard 2014; Posel et al. 2014). Most approaches pertain to education in the clinical workplace. Box 1.3 gives a condensed overview.

One dominant approach that clinical educators use when teaching students to solve medical problems is ask them to analyze pathophysiologically, in other words to use System 2 thinking. While this seems the only option with students who do not

---

Box 1.3 Summary of Recommended Approaches to Teaching Clinical Reasoning (Guerrasio and Aagaard 2014; Rencic 2011; Posel et al. 2014; Chamberland et al. 2015; Balslev et al. 2015; Bowen 2006)

Let students

- Maximize learning by remembering many patient encounters.
- Recall similar cases as they increase experience.
- Build a framework for differential diagnosis using anatomy, pathology, and organ systems combined with semantic qualifiers: age, gender, ethnicity, and main complaint.
- Differentiate between likely and less likely but important diagnoses.
- Contrast diagnoses by listing necessary history questions and physical exam maneuvers in a tabular format and indicating what supports or does not support the respective diagnoses.
- Utilize epidemiology, evidence, and Bayesian reasoning.
- Practice deliberately; request and reflect on feedback; and practice mentally.
- Generate self-explanations during clinical problem solving.
- Talk in buzz groups at morning reports with oral and written patient data.
- Listen to clinical teachers reasoning out loud.
- Summarize clinical cases often using semantic qualifiers and create problem representations.

possess a mental library of illness scripts to facilitate System 1 thinking, those teachers teach something they usually do not do themselves when solving clinical problems This teaching resembles the "do as I say, not as I do" approach, in part because they simply cannot express "how they do" when they engaged in clinical reasoning.

In a recent review of approaches to the teaching of clinical reasoning, Schmidt and Mamede identified two groups of approaches: a predominant serial-cue approach (teachers provide bits of patient information to students and ask them to reason step by step) and a rare whole-task (or whole-case) approach in which all information is presented at once. They conclude that there is little evidence for the serial-cue approach, favored by most teachers and recommend a switch to whole-case approaches (Schmidt and Mamede 2015). While cognitive theory does support whole-task instructional techniques (Vandewaetere et al. 2014), the description of a whole-case in clinical education is not well elaborated. Evidently a whole-case cannot include a diagnosis and must at least be partly serial. But even if all the information that clinicians in practice face is provided to students all at once, the clinical reasoning process that follows has a serial nature, even if it happens quickly. Schmidt and Mamede's proposal to first develop causal explanations, second to encapsulate pathophysiological knowledge, and third to develop illness scripts (Schmidt and Mamede 2015) runs the risk of separating biomedical knowledge acquisition from clinical training and regressing to a Flexnerian curriculum. Flexner advocated a strong biomedical background before students start dealing with patients (Flexner 1910). This separation is currently not considered the most useful approach to clinical reasoning education (Woods 2007; Chamberland et al. 2013).

Training students in the skill of clinical reasoning is evidently a difficult task, and Schuwirth rightly once posed the question "Can clinical reasoning be taught or can it only be learned?" (Schuwirth 2002). Since the work of Elstein and colleagues, we know that clinical reasoning is not a skill that is trainable independent of a large knowledge base (Elstein et al. 1978). There simply is not an effective and teachable algorithm of clinical problem solving that can be trained and learned, if there is no medical knowledge base. The actual reasoning techniques used in clinical problem solving can be explained rather briefly and may not be very different from those of a car mechanic. Listen to the patient (or the car owner), examine the patient (or the car), draw conclusions, and identify what it takes to solve the problem. There is not much more to it. In difficult cases, medical decision-making can require knowledge of Bayesian probability calculations, understanding of sensitivity and specificity of tests (Kassirer et al. 2010), but clinicians seldom use these advanced techniques explicitly at the bedside.

These recommendations are of no avail if students do not have background knowledge, both about anatomical structures and pathophysiological processes and about patterns of signs and symptoms related to illness scripts. When training medical students to think like doctors, we face the problem that we cannot just look how clinicians think and just ask students to mimic that technique. That is for two reasons: one is that clinicians often cannot express well how they think, and the second is simply that the huge knowledge base required to think like an experienced clinician is simply not present in students.

As System 1 pattern recognition is so overwhelmingly dominant in the clinician's thinking (Norman et al. 2007), the lack of a knowledge base prohibits junior students to think like a doctor. It is clear that students cannot "recognize" a pattern if they do not have a similar pattern in their knowledge base. It is unavoidable that much effort and extensive experience are needed before a reasonable repository of illness scripts is built that can serve as the internal mirror of patterns seen in clinical practice. Ericsson's work suggests that it may take up to 10,000 hours of deliberate practice to acquire expertise in any domain, although there is some debate about this volume (Ericsson et al. 1993; Macnamara et al. 2014). Clearly, students must see and experience many, many cases and construct and remember illness scripts. What a curriculum can try to offer is just that, i.e., many clinical encounters, in clinical settings or in a simulated environment. Clinical context is likely to enhance clinical knowledge, specifically if students feel a sense of responsibility or commitment (Koens et al. 2005; Koens 2005). This sense of commitment in practice relates to the patient, but it can also be a commitment to teach peers.

System 2 analytic reasoning is clearly a skill that *can* be trained early in a curriculum (Ploger 1988). Causal reasoning, usually starting with pathology (a viral infection of the liver) and a subsequent effect (preventing the draining of red blood cell waste products) and ending with resulting symptoms (yellow stains in the blood, visible in the sclerae of the eyes and in the skin, known as jaundice or icterus), can be understood and remembered, and the reasoning can include deeper biochemical or microbiological explanations (How does it operate the chemical degradation of hemoglobin? Which viruses cause hepatitis? How was the patient infected?). This basically is a systems-based reasoning process. The clinician however must reason in the opposite direction, a skill that is not simply the reverse of this chain of thought, as there may be very different causes of the same signs and symptoms (a normal liver, but an obstruction in the bile duct, or a normal liver and bile duct, but a profuse destruction of red blood cells after an immune reaction). So analytic reasoning is trainable, and generating hypotheses of what may have caused the symptoms requires a knowledge base of possible physiopathology mechanisms. That can be acquired step by step, and many answers to analytic problems can be found in the literature. But clearly, System 2 reasoning too requires prior knowledge. So both a basic science knowledge base and a mental illness script repository must be available.

The case-based clinical reasoning training method acknowledges this difficulty and therefore focuses on two simultaneous approaches (1) building illness scripts from early on in the curriculum, beginning with simple cases and gradually building more complex scripts to remember, and (2) conveying a systematic, analytic reasoning habit starting with patient presentation vignettes and ending with a conclusion about the diagnosis, the disease mechanism, and the patient management actions to be taken.

Summary of the CBCR Method

When applying these principles to preclinical classroom teaching, a case-based approach is considered superior to other methods (Kim et al. 2006; Postma and White 2015). Case-based clinical reasoning was designed at the Academic Medical Center of University of Amsterdam in 1992, when a new undergraduate medical curriculum was introduced (ten Cate and Schadé 1993; ten Cate 1994, 1995). This integrated medical curriculum with multidisciplinary block modules of 6–8 weeks had existed since 10 years, but was found to lack a proper preparation of students to think like a doctor before entering clinical clerkships. Notably, while all block modules stressed the knowledge acquisition structured in a systematic way, usually based on organ systems and resulting in a systems knowledge base, a longitudinal thread of small group teaching was created to focus on patient-oriented thinking, with application of acquired knowledge (ten Cate and Schadé 1993). This CBCR training was implemented in curriculum years 2, 3, and 4, at both medical schools of the University of Amsterdam and the Free University of Amsterdam, which had been collaborating on curriculum development since the late 1980s. After an explanation of the method in national publications (ten Cate 1994, 1995), medical schools at Leiden and Rotterdam universities adopted variants of it. In 1997 CBCR was introduced at the medical school of Utrecht University with minor modifications and continued with only little adaptations throughout major undergraduate medical curriculum changes in 1999, 2006, and 2015 until the current day (2017).

CBCR can be summarized as the practicing of clinical reasoning in small groups. A CBCR course consists of a series of group sessions over a prolonged time span. This may be a semester, a year, or usually, a number of years. Students regularly meet in a fixed group of 10–12, usually every 3–4 weeks, but this may be more frequent. The course is independent of concurrent courses or blocks. The rationale for this is that CBCR stresses the application of previously acquired knowledge and should not be programmed as an "illustration" of clinical or basic science theory. More importantly, when the case starts, students must not be cued in specific directions or diagnoses, which would be the case if a session were integrated in, say, a cardiovascular block. A patient with shortness of breath would then trigger too easily toward a cardiac problem.

CBCR cases, always titled with age, sex, and main complaint or symptom, consist of an introductory case vignette reflecting the way a patient presents at the clinician's office. Alternatively, two cases with similar presentations but different diagnoses may be worked through in one session, usually later in the curriculum when the thinking process can be speeded up. The context of the case may be at a general practitioner's office, at an emergency department, at an outpatient clinic, or at admission to a hospital ward. The case vignette continues with questions and assignments (e.g., *What would be first hypotheses based on the information so far? What diagnostic tests should be ordered? Draw a table mapping signs and symptoms against likelihood of hypotheses*), at fixed moments interrupted with the provision of new findings about the patient from investigations (more extensive history, additional physical examination, or new results of diagnostic tests), distributed or read out loud by a facilitator during the session at the appropriate moment. A full case includes the complete course of a problem from the initial presentation to follow-up after treatment, but cases often concentrate on key stages of this course. Case descriptions should refer to relevant pathophysiological backgrounds and basic sciences (such as anatomy, biochemistry, cell biology, physiology) during the case.

The sessions are led by three (sometimes two) students of the group. They are called *peer teachers* and take turns in this role over the whole course. Every student must act as a peer teacher at multiple sessions across the year. Peer teachers have more information in advance about the patient and disclose this information at the appropriate time during the session, in accordance with instructions they receive in advance. In addition, a clinician is present. Given the elaborated format and case description, this teacher only acts as a consultant, when guidance is requested or helpful, and indeed is called "consultant" throughout all CBCR education.

Study materials include a general study guide with explanations of the rules, courses of action, assessment procedures, etc. (see Chap. 10): a "student version" of the written CBCR case material per session, a "peer teacher version" of the CBCR case per session with extra information and hints to guide the group, and a full "consultant version" of the CBCR case per session. Short handouts are also available for all students, covering new clinical information when needed in the course of the diagnostic process. Optionally, homemade handouts can be prepared by peer teachers. The full consultant version of the CBCR case includes all answers to all questions in detail, sufficient to enable guidance by a clinician who is not familiar with the case or discipline, all suggestions and hints for peer teachers, and all patient information that should be disclosed during the session. Examples are shown in Appendices of this book.

Students are assessed at the end of the course on their knowledge of all illnesses and to a small extent on their active participation as a student and a peer teacher (see Chap. 7).

Essential Features of CBCR Education

While a summary is given above, and a detailed procedural description is given in Part II, it may be helpful to provide some principles to help understand some of the rationale behind the CBCR method.

Switching Between System-Oriented Thinking and Patient-Oriented Thinking

It is our belief that preclinical students must learn to acquire both system-oriented knowledge and patient-oriented knowledge and that they need to practice switching between both modes of thinking (Eva et al. 2007). In that sense, our approach not only differs from traditional curricula with no training in clinical reasoning but also from curricula in which all education is derived from clinical presentations (Mandin et al. 1995, 1997).

By scheduling CBCR sessions spread over the year, with each session requiring the clinical application of system knowledge of previous system courses, this practice of switching is stimulated. It is important to prepare and schedule CBCR cases carefully to enable this knowledge application. It is inevitable, because of differential diagnostic thinking, that cases draw upon knowledge from different courses and sometimes knowledge that may not have been taught. In that case, additional information may be provided during the case discussion. Peer teachers often have an assignment to summarize relevant system information between case questions in a brief presentation (maximum 10 min), to enable further progression.

Managing Cognitive Load and the Development of Illness Scripts

Illness scripts are mental representations of disease entities combining three elements in a script (Custers et al. 1998; Charlin et al. 2007): (1) factors causing or preceding a disease, (2) the actual pathology, and (3) the effect of the pathology showing as signs, symptoms, and expected diagnostic findings. While some authors, including us, add (4) course and management as the fourth element (de Vries et al. 2006), originally the first three, "enabling conditions," "fault," and "consequences," were proposed to constitute the illness script (Feltovich and Barrows 1984). Illness scripts are stored as units in the long-term memory that are simultaneously activated and subsequently instantiated (i.e., recalled instantly) when a pattern recognition process occurs based on a patient seen by a doctor. This process is usually not deliberately executed, but occurs spontaneously. Illness scripts have a temporal nature like a film script, because of their cause and effect features, which enables clinicians to quickly take a next step, suggested by the script, in managing the patient. "Course and management" can therefore naturally be considered part of the script.

A shared explanation why illness scripts "work" in clinical reasoning is that the human working memory is very limited and does not allow to process much more than seven units or *chunks* of information at a time (Miller 1956) and likely less than that. Clinicians cannot process all separate signs and symptoms, history, and physical examination information simultaneously—that would overload their working memory capacity, but try to use one label to combine many bits of information in one unit (e.g., the illness script "diabetes type II" combines its enabling factors, pathology, signs and symptoms, disease course, and standard treatment in one chunk). If necessary, those units can be unpacked in elements (Figs. 1.1 and 1.2).

To create illness scripts stored in the long-term memory, students must learn to see illnesses as a unit of information. In case-based clinical reasoning education,

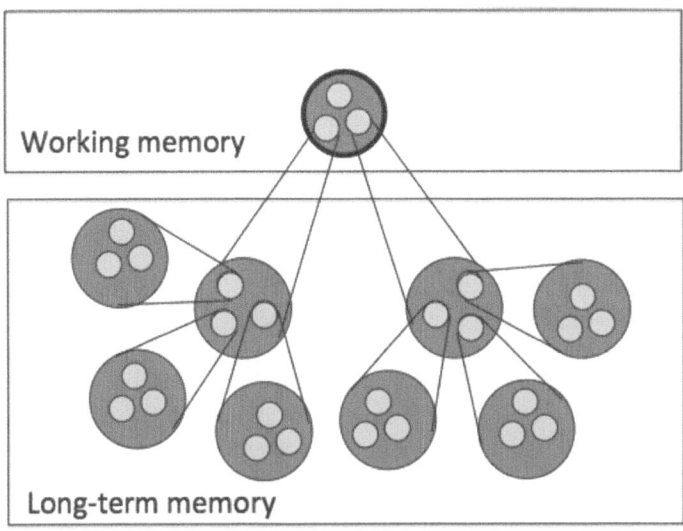

Fig. 1.2 One information chunk in the working memory may be decomposed in smaller chunks in the long-term memory (Young et al. 2014)

students face complete patient scripts, i.e., with enabling conditions (often derived from history taking) to consequences (as presenting signs and symptoms). Although illness scripts have an implicit chronology, from a clinical reasoning perspective, there is an adapted chronology of (a) consequences → (b) enabling conditions → (c) fault and diagnosis → (d) course and management, as the physician starts out observing the signs and symptoms, then takes a history, performs a physical examination, and orders tests if necessary before arriving at a conclusion about the "fault." To enable building illness script units in the long-term memory, students must start out with simple, prototype cases that can be easily remembered. CBCR aims to develop in second year medical students stable but still somewhat limited illness scripts. This still limited repository should be sufficient to quickly recognize the causes, symptoms, and management of a limited series of common illnesses, and handle prototypical patient problems in practice if they would encounter these, resonating with Bordage's prototype approach (Bordage and Zacks 1984; Bordage 2007). See Chap. 3. The assessment of student knowledge at the end of a CBCR course focuses on the exact cases discussed, including, of course, the differential diagnostic considerations that are activated with the illness script, all to reinforce the same carefully chosen illness scripts. The aim is to provide a foundation that enables the addition in later years of variations to the prototypical cases learned, to enrich further illness script formation and from there add new illness scripts. We believe that working with whole, but not too complex, cases in an early phase in the medical curriculum serves to help students in an early phase in the medical curriculum to learn to recognize common patterns.

Educational Philosophies: Active Reasoning by Oral Communication and Peer Teaching

A CBCR education in the format elaborated in this book reflects the philosophy that learning clinical reasoning is enhanced by reasoning aloud. The small group arrangement, limited to no more than about 12 students, guarantees that every student actively contributes to the discussion. Even when listening, this group size precludes from hiding as would be a risk in a lecture setting.

Students act as peer teachers for their fellow students. Peer teaching is an accepted educational method with a theoretical foundation (ten Cate and Durning 2007; Topping 1996). It is well known that taking the role of teacher for peers stimulates knowledge acquisition in a different and often more productive way than studying for an exam (Bargh and Schul 1980). Social and cognitive congruence concepts explain why students benefit from communicating with peers or near-peers and should understand each other better than when students communicate with expert teachers (Lockspeiser et al. 2008). The peer teaching format used in CBCR is an excellent way to achieve active participation of all students during small group education. An additional benefit of using peer teachers is that they are instrumental in the provision of just-in-time information about the clinical case for their peers in the CBCR group, e.g., as a result of a diagnostic test that was proposed to be ordered.

Case-based clinical reasoning has most of the features that are recommended by Kassirer et al.: "First, clinical data are presented, analyzed and discussed in the same chronological sequence in which they were obtained in the course of the encounter between the physician and the patient. Second, instead of providing all available data completely synthesized in one cohesive story, as is in the practice of the traditional case presentation, data are provided and considered on a little at a time. Third, any cases presented should consist of real, unabridged patient material. Simulated cases or modified actual cases should be avoided because they may fail to reflect the true inconsistencies, false leads, inappropriate cues, and fuzzy data inherent in actual patient material. Finally, the careful selection of examples of problem solving ensures that a reasonable set of cognitive concepts will be covered" (Kassirer et al. 2010). While we agree with the third condition for advanced students, i.e., in clerkship years, for pre-clerkship medical students, a prototypical illness script is considered more appropriate and effective (Bordage 2007). The CBCR method also matches well with most recommendations on clinical reasoning education (see Box 1.3).

Chapter 4 of this book describes six prerequisites for clinical reasoning by medical students in the clinical context: having clinical vocabulary, experience with problem representation, an illness script mental repository, a contrastive learning approach, hypothesis-driven inquiry skill, and a habit of diagnostic verification. The CBCR approach helps to prepare students with most of these prerequisites.

Indications for the Effectiveness of the CBCR Method

The CBCR method finds its roots in part in problem-based learning (PBL) and other small group active learning approaches. Since the 1970s, various small group approaches have been recommended for medical education, notably PBL (Barrows and Tamblyn 1980) and team-based learning (TBL) (Michaelsen et al. 2008). In particular PBL has gained huge interest in the 1980s onward, due to the developmental work done by its founder Howard Barrows from McMaster University in Canada and from Maastricht University in the Netherlands, which institution derived its entire identity to a large part from problem-based learning. Despite significant research efforts to establish the superiority of PBL curricula, the general outcomes have been somewhat less than expected (Dolmans and Gijbels 2013). However, many studies on a more detailed level have shown that components of PBL are effective. In a recent overviews of PBL studies, Dolmans and Wilkerson conclude that "a clearly formulated problem, an especially socially congruent tutor, a cognitive congruent tutor with expertise, and a focused group discussion have a strong influence on students' learning and achievement" (Dolmans and Wilkerson 2011). These are components that are included in the CBCR method.

While there has not been a controlled study to establish the effect of a CBCR course per se, compared to an alternative approach to clinical reasoning training, there is some indirect support for its validity, apart from the favorable reception of the teaching model among clinicians and students over the course of 20 years and different schools. A recent publication by Krupat and colleagues showed that a "case-based collaborative learning" format, including small group work on patient cases with sequential provision of patient information, led to higher scores of a physiology exam and high appreciation among students, compared with education using a problem-based learning format (Krupat et al. 2016). A more indirect indication of its effectiveness is shown in a comparative study among three schools in the Netherlands two decades ago (Schmidt et al. 1996). One of the schools, the University of Amsterdam medical school, had used the CBCR training among second and third year students at that time (ten Cate 1994). While the study does not specifically report on the effects of clinical reasoning education, Schmidt et al. show how students of the second and third year in this curriculum outperform students in both other curricula in diagnostic competence.

CBCR as an Approach to Ignite Curriculum Modernization

Since 2005, the method of CBCR has been used as leverage for undergraduate medical curriculum reform in Moldova, Georgia, Ukraine, and Azerbaijan (ten Cate et al. 2014). It has proven to be useful in medical education contexts with heavily lecture-based curricula—likely because the method can be applied within an existing curriculum, causing little disruption, while also being exemplary for recommended modern medical education (Harden et al. 1984). It stimulates integration, and the method is highly student-centered and problem-based. While observing CBCR in practice, a school can consider how these features can also be applied more generally in preclinical courses. This volume provides a detailed description that allows a school to pilot CBCR for this purpose.

References

Audétat, M.-C., et al. (2013). Clinical reasoning difficulties: A taxonomy for clinical teachers. *Medical Teacher, 35*(3), e984–e989. Available at: http://www.ncbi.nlm.nih.gov/pubmed/23228082.

Balogh, E. P., Miller, B. T., & Ball, J. R. (2015). *Improving diagnosis in healthcare*. Washington, DC: The Institute of Medicine and the National Academies Press. Available at: http://www.nap.edu/catalog/21794/improving-diagnosis-in-health-care.

Balslev, T., et al. (2015). Combining bimodal presentation schemes and buzz groups improves clinical reasoning and learning at morning report. *Medical Teacher, 37*(8), 759–766. Available at: http://informahealthcare.com/doi/abs/10.3109/0142159X.2014.986445.

Bargh, J. A., & Schul, Y. (1980). On the cognitive benefits of teaching. *Journal of Educational Psychology, 72*(5), 593–604.

Barrows, H. S., & Tamblyn, R. M. (1980). *Problem-based learning. An approach to medical education*. New York: Springer.

Bordage, G. (2007). Prototypes and semantic qualifiers: From past to present. *Medical Education, 41*(12), 1117–1121.

Bordage, G., & Zacks, R. (1984). The structure of medical knowledge in the memories of medical students and general practitioners: Categories and prototypes. *Medical Education, 18*(11), 406–416.

Boshuizen, H., & Schmidt, H. (2000). The development of clinical reasoning expertise. In J. Higg & M. Jones (Eds.), *Clinical reasoning in the health professions* (pp. 15–22). Butterworth Heinemann: Oxford.

Bowen, J. L. (2006). Educational strategies to promote clinical diagnostic reasoning. *The New England Journal of Medicine, 355*(21), 2217–2225.

Chamberland, M., et al. (2013). Students' self-explanations while solving unfamiliar cases: The role of biomedical knowledge. *Medical Education, 47*(11), 1109–1116.

Chamberland, M., et al. (2015). Self-explanation in learning clinical reasoning: The added value of examples and prompts. *Medical Education, 49*, 193–202.

Charlin, B., et al. (2007). Scripts and clinical reasoning. *Medical Education, 41*(12), 1178–1184.

Croskerry, P. (2009). A universal model of diagnostic reasoning. *Academic Medicine: Journal of the Association of American Medical Colleges, 84*(8), 1022–1028.

Custers, E. J. F. M. (2013). Medical education and cognitive continuum theory: An alternative perspective on medical problem solving and clinical reasoning. *Academic Medicine, 88*(8), 1074–1080.

Custers, E. J. F. M., Boshuizen, H. P. A., & Schmidt, H. G. (1998). The role of illness scripts in the development of medical diagnostic expertise: Results from an interview study. *Cognition and Instruction, 14*(4), 367–398.

de Vries, A., Custers, E., & ten Cate, O. (2006). Teaching clinical reasoning and the development of illness scripts: Possibilities in medical education. [Dutch]. *Dutch Journal of Medical Education, 25*(1), 2–2.

Dolmans, D., & Gijbels, D. (2013). Research on problem-based learning: Future challenges. *Medical Education, 47*(2), 214–218. Available at: http://www.ncbi.nlm.nih.gov/pubmed/23323661. Accessed 26 May 2013.

Dolmans, D. H. J. M., & Wilkerson, L. (2011). Reflection on studies on the learning process in problem-based learning. *Advances in Health Sciences Education: Theory and Practice, 16*(4), 437–441. Available at: http://www.pubmedcentral.nih.gov/articlerender.fcgi?artid=3166125&tool=pmcentrez&rendertype=abstract. Accessed 11 Mar 2012.

Elstein, A. (1995). Clinical reasoning in medicine. In J. Higgs & M. Jones (Eds.), *Clinical reasoning in the health professions* (pp. 49–59). Oxford: Butterworth Heinemann.

Elstein, A. S., Shulman, L. S., & Sprafka, S. A. (1978). Medical problem solving. In *An analysis of clinical reasoning*. Cambridge, MA: Harvard University Press.

Ericsson, K. A., et al. (1993). The role of deliberate practice in the acquisition of expert performance. *Psychological Review, 100*(3), 363–406.

Eva, K. W. (2005). What every teacher needs to know about clinical reasoning. *Medical Education, 39*(1), 98–106.

Eva, K. W., et al. (2007). Teaching from the clinical reasoning literature: Combined reasoning strategies help novice diagnosticians overcome misleading information. *Medical Education, 41*(12), 1152–1158.

Feltovich, P., & Barrows, H. (1984). Issues of generality in medical problem solving. In H. G. Schmidt & M. L. de Voider (Eds.), *Tutorials in problem-based learning* (pp. 128–170). Assen: Van Gorcum.

Flexner, A., 1910. *Medical Education in the United States and Canada. A report to the Carnegie Foundation for the Advancement of Teaching*. Repr. ForgottenBooks. Boston: D.B. Updike, the Merrymount Press.

Graber, M. L., Franklin, N., & Gordon, R. (2005). Diagnostic error in internal medicine. *Archives of Internal Medicine, 165*(13), 1493–1499.

Guerrasio, J., & Aagaard, E. M. (2014). Methods and outcomes for the remediation of clinical reasoning. *Journal of General Internal Medicine*, 1607–1614.

Harden, R. M., Sowden, S., & Dunn, W. (1984). Educational strategies in curriculum development: The SPICES model. *Medical Education, 18*, 284–297.

Higgs, J., & Jones, M. (2000). In J. Higgs & M. Jones (Eds.), *Clinical reasoning in the health professions* (2nd ed.). Woburn: Butterworth-Heinemann.

Hruska, P., et al. (2015). Hemispheric activation differences in novice and expert clinicians during clinical decision making. *Advances in Health Sciences Education, 21*, 1–13.

Kahneman, D., & Klein, G. (2009). Conditions for intuitive expertise: A failure to disagree. *The American Psychologist, 64*(6), 515–526.

Kassirer, J. P. (2010). Teaching clinical reasoning: Case-based and coached. *Academic Medicine, 85*(7), 1118–1124.

Kassirer, J., Wong, J., & Kopelman, R. (2010). *Learning clinical reasoning* (2nd ed.). Baltimore: Lippincott Williams & Wilkins.

Kim, S., et al. (2006). A conceptual framework for developing teaching cases: A review and synthesis of the literature across disciplines. *Medical Education, 40*(9), 867–876.

Koens, F. (2005). *Vertical integration in medical education*. Doctoral dissertation, Utrecht University, Utrecht.

Koens, F., et al. (2005). Analysing the concept of context in medical education. *Medical Education, 39*(12), 1243–1249.

Krupat, E., et al. (2016). Assessing the effectiveness of case-based collaborative learning via randomized controlled trial. *Academic Medicine, 91(5), 723–729*.

Lee, A., et al. (2010). Using illness scripts to teach clinical reasoning skills to medical students. *Family Medicine, 42*(4), 255–261.

Lockspeiser, T. M., et al. (2008). Understanding the experience of being taught by peers: The value of social and cognitive congruence. *Advances in Health Sciences Education: Theory and Practice, 13*(3), 361–372.

Macnamara, B. N., Hambrick, D. Z., & Oswald, F. L. (2014). Deliberate practice and performance in music, games, sports, education, and professions: A meta-analysis. *Psychological Science, 24*(8), 1608–1618.

Mandin, H., et al. (1995). Developing a "clinical presentation" curriculum at the University of Calgary. *Academic Medicine, 70*(3), 186–193.

Mandin, H., et al. (1997). Helping students learn to think like experts when solving clinical problems. *Academic Medicine, 72*(3), 173–179.

McGlynn, E. A., McDonald, K. M., & Cassel, C. K. (2015). Measurement is essential for improving diagnosis and reducing diagnostic error. *JAMA, 314*, 1.

Michaelsen, L., et al. (2008). *Team-based learning for health professions education.* Sterling: Stylus Publishing, LLC.

Miller, G. A. (1956). The magical number seven, plus or minus two: Some limits on our capacity for processing information. *Psychological Review, 63*, 81–97.

Norman, G., Young, M., & Brooks, L. (2007). Non-analytical models of clinical reasoning: The role of experience. *Medical Education, 41*(12), 1140–1145.

Norman, G., et al. (2014). The etiology of diagnostic errors: A controlled trial of system 1 versus system 2 reasoning. *Academic Medicine: Journal of the Association of American Medical Colleges, 89*(2), 277–284.

Norman, G. R., et al. (2017). The causes of errors in clinical reasoning: Cognitive biases, knowledge deficits, and dual process thinking. *Academic Medicine, 92*(1), 23–30.

Pelaccia, T., et al. (2011). An analysis of clinical reasoning through a recent and comprehensive approach: The dual-process theory. *Medical Education Online, 16*, 1–9.

Ploger, D. (1988). Reasoning and the structure of knowledge in biochemistry. *Instructional Science, 17*(1988), 57–76.

Posel, N., Mcgee, J. B., & Fleiszer, D. M. (2014). Twelve tips to support the development of clinical reasoning skills using virtual patient cases. *Medical Teacher, 0*(0), 1–6.

Postma, T. C., & White, J. G. (2015). Developing clinical reasoning in the classroom – Analysis of the 4C/ID-model. *European Journal of Dental Education, 19*(2), 74–80.

Rencic, J. (2011). Twelve tips for teaching expertise in clinical reasoning. *Medical Teacher, 33*(11), 887–892. Available at: http://www.ncbi.nlm.nih.gov/pubmed/21711217. Accessed 1 Mar 2012.

Schmidt, H. (1983). Problem-based learning: Rationale and description. *Medical Education, 17*(1), 11–16.

Schmidt, H. G., & Mamede, S. (2015). How to improve the teaching of clinical reasoning: A narrative review and a proposal. *Medical Education, 49*(10), 961–973.

Schmidt, H., et al. (1996). The development of diagnostic competence: Comparison of a problem-based, and integrated and a conventional medical curriculum. *Academic Medicine, 71*(6), 658–664.

Schuwirth, L. (2002). Can clinical reasoning be taught or can it only be learned? *Medical Education, 36*(8), 695–696.

ten Cate, T. J. (1994). Training case-based clinical reasoning in small groups [Dutch]. *Nederlands Tijdschrift voor Geneeskunde, 138*, 1238–1243.

ten Cate, T. J. (1995). Teaching small groups [Dutch]. In J. Metz, A. Scherpbier, & C. Van der Vleuten (Eds.), *Medical education in practice* (pp. 45–57). Assen: Van Gorcum.

ten Cate, T. J., & Schadé, E. (1993). Workshops clinical decision-making. One year experience with small group case-based clinical reasoning education. In J. Metz, A. Scherpbier, & E. Houtkoop (Eds.), *Gezond Onderwijs 2 – proceedings of the second national conference on medical education [Dutch]* (pp. 215–222). Nijmegen: Universitair Publikatiebureau KUN.

ten Cate, O., & Durning, S. (2007). Dimensions and psychology of peer teaching in medical education. *Medical Teacher, 29*(6), 546–552.

ten Cate, O., Van Loon, M., & Simonia, G. (Eds.). (2014). *Modernizing medical education through case-based clinical reasoning* (1st ed.). Utrecht: University Medical Center Utrecht. with translations in Georgian, Ukrainian, Azeri and Spanish.

Topping, K. J. (1996). The effectiveness of peer tutoring in further and higher education: A typology and review of the literature. *Higher Education, 32*, 321–345.

Vandewaetere, M., et al. (2014). 4C/ID in medical education: How to design an educational program based on whole-task learning: AMEE guide no. 93. *Medical Teacher, 93*, 1–17.

Williams, R. G., et al. (2011). Tracking development of clinical reasoning ability across five medical schools using a progress test. *Academic Medicine: Journal of the Association of American Medical Colleges, 86*(9), 1148–1154.

Woods, N. N. (2007). Science is fundamental: The role of biomedical knowledge in clinical reasoning. *Medical Education, 41*(12), 1173–1177.

Young, J. Q., et al. (2014). Cognitive load theory: Implications for medical education: AMEE guide no. 86. *Medical Teacher, 36*(5), 371–384.

Open Access This chapter is licensed under the terms of the Creative Commons Attribution 4.0 International License (http://creativecommons.org/licenses/by/4.0/), which permits use, sharing, adaptation, distribution and reproduction in any medium or format, as long as you give appropriate credit to the original author(s) and the source, provide a link to the Creative Commons license and indicate if changes were made.

The images or other third party material in this chapter are included in the chapter's Creative Commons license, unless indicated otherwise in a credit line to the material. If material is not included in the chapter's Creative Commons license and your intended use is not permitted by statutory regulation or exceeds the permitted use, you will need to obtain permission directly from the copyright holder.

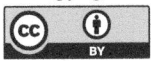

Chapter 2
Training Clinical Reasoning: Historical and Theoretical Background

Eugène J.F.M. Custers

In this chapter, we will try to give a concise overview of what is known about teaching clinical reasoning in the era before the concept of "clinical reasoning" as such emerged in the literature. Not surprisingly, the further we go back in time, the more this concept needs to be stretched to fit what can arguably be seen as the predecessors of today's clinical teaching and diagnostic reasoning. Yet, even in the earliest days of medicine, teachers taught students how to make sense of the findings associated with diseases (patients' complaints, signs, and symptoms) and how to use this knowledge to ameliorate a patient's condition, if this could be achieved at all. Starting in the 1950s, clinical reasoning itself became a subject of study, which increasingly enabled clinical educators to advance beyond merely showing and telling students how to apply knowledge and skills in a practical setting, to building theories and models of how clinical reasoning can be effectively and efficiently trained.

Clinical Reasoning in the Hippocratean Era

Through all ages, humans have tried to make sense of complaints, symptoms, and diseases; in this sense, clinical reasoning is as old as humanity. In the pre-Hippocratic era, people relied on priests or other authoritative individuals who had privileged access to the intentions divine entities had with the sufferer or with society as a whole, for diseases were sometimes seen – by patients as well as by healers – as containing messages from above. Similarly, the cause of a disease could be couched

---

E.J.F.M. Custers (✉)
Center for Research and Development of Education, University Medical Center Utrecht, Utrecht, The Netherlands
e-mail: E.J.F.M.Custers@umcutrecht.nl

© The Authors 2018
O. ten Cate et al. (eds.), *Principles and Practice of Case-based Clinical Reasoning Education*, Innovation and Change in Professional Education 15, https://doi.org/10.1007/978-3-319-64828-6_2

in moral terms, and symptoms and complaints were interpreted as punishment or revenge, from the part of the gods, for the sufferer's misbehavior. As far as we know, Hippocrates (± 460 BC – ± 370 BC) was the first to acknowledge the natural, i.e., non-divine, nature of diseases. That is, he explained disease in terms of a disturbance of the balance of the four humors: yellow bile, black bile, blood, and phlegm, an explanation that was further elaborated by Galen (131–216) and, though lacking a firm empirical basis, was so convincing that it remained basically unchallenged for two millennia. With respect to treatment, nature itself was assumed to have healing powers, and therapeutic measures aimed at supporting these natural forces. Probably the biggest contributions of Hippocrates and Galen to clinical reasoning was their emphasis on careful observation and registration of all visible symptoms and complaints, including bodily fluids and excretions, as well as environmental factors, diet, and living habits. Hippocrates summarized much of his practical knowledge in aphorisms, many of which are rules of thumb in the "if… then" format. Such rules of thumb, or heuristics, can be viewed as a rudimentary form of clinical reasoning. Though most Hippocratean aphorisms deal with treatment or prediction of the course of an illness, some are about diagnosis (e.g., "In those cases where there is a sandy sediment in the urine, there is calculus in the bladder or kidneys"). The aphorisms were largely based on experience, rather than "logically" derived from Hippocratean humoral theory. In fact, this disconnection between disease theory and clinical practice remained intact until well into the nineteenth century, when methods were developed to investigate the inner workings of the living human body. Even in today's clinical reasoning, aphorism-like heuristics still play an important role in the diagnostic process (e.g., "if symptom X, then always consider disease Y"), though nowadays generally supported by knowledge of underlying biomedical and pathophysiological mechanisms (Becker et al. 1961; Mangrulkar et al. 2002; Sanders 2009).

Bedside Teaching and Patient Demonstration

Until well into the seventeenth century, academic medicine was almost exclusively a theoretical affair. Reasoning played an important role, but it was exclusively employed to defend theses or to construct logical arguments, rather than to arrive at diagnoses or to select therapies. The introduction of bedside teaching by Batista de Monte in Padua in 1543 may have been the first step in teaching clinical reasoning in a more empirical sense, though little is known about his actual teaching and it was already discontinued by his immediate successors. Attempts to introduce bedside teaching in the Netherlands by Willem van der Straaten in Utrecht (1636) and Jan Van Heurne in Leyden (1638) met a similar fate. Herman Boerhaave (1668–1738) at Leyden University was more successful, and his "model" was followed by Edinburgh and Vienna, from where it spread to other universities in Europe and North America. Yet, even at Boerhaave's department, this form of teaching played only a marginal role, largely due to lack of access to suitable patients. Moreover,

Boerhaave's bedside teachings were in fact orchestrated patient demonstrations, rather than sessions in which clinical reasoning was taught. Boerhaave's aim was to achieve an integration, in his students, of theoretical knowledge from books and lectures – "advanced Hippocratean and Galenic theory" – and clinical experience (Risse 1989).

An important next step was made in 1766. In this year, Dr. Thomas Bond delivered his *Introductory Lecture to a Course of Clinical Observations in the Pennsylvania Hospital*, at the first medical school in America, the Medical College of the University of Pennsylvania. Bond was probably the first teacher to have unrestricted access to a sizeable number of patients in the hospital wards (Flexner 1910) (p. 4). Bond also appears to be the first teacher who introduced empirical elements into the – until then theoretically closed – system of clinical reasoning. That is, unlike Boerhaave's, Bond's reasoning could end in predictions that could conflict with empirical observations at obduction. If a patient had died, Bond predicted, rather than just demonstrated, the findings at autopsy. He was well aware of the risk that his predictions were not necessarily borne out: "...if perchance he [the teacher] finds [at autopsy] something unsuspected, which betrays an error in judgment, he like a great and good man, immediately acknowledges the mistake, and for the benefit of survivors points out other methods by which it might have been more hapily treated" (Bridenbaugh 1947) (p. 14). By exposing his clinical reasoning to empirical refutation, Bond opened the door to actual improvement of this reasoning and, as a corollary, to better understanding of the relationship between visible pathology and disease, with the possibility of improving treatment as well.

William Osler and the Differential Diagnosis

Basically, the early nineteenth century saw a rapid abandonment of Hippocratean-Galenic medical theory in favor of modern scientific medicine, which conceives of diseases as derailments of normal processes (or normal structures), rather than as disturbances of some speculative form of homeostasis. New diagnostic tools became available, such as palpation, percussion, and auscultation, which enabled the physician to investigate the interior of the human body without opening it and to distinguish between normal functioning (or structures) and their pathological deviations. The task of the clinician gradually shifted from accurate description of symptoms to drawing conclusions, on basis of indirect information, about underlying pathophysiological or pathological processes. Diseases were no longer defined exclusively on basis of findings (complaints, signs, and symptoms), and it was acknowledged that different diseases could lead to similar symptoms. This led to the emergence of the concept of a differential diagnosis. William Osler (1849–1919) is not only viewed as the founder of North-American clinical medicine, but he is also credited with introducing the "discipline of differential diagnosis" (Maude 2014). A differential diagnosis is a necessary concept if one wants to approach clinical problem solving in a systematic way, taking into account different possible causes of a particular symptom.

Abraham Flexner and the Science of Clinical Medicine

The reformer of American medical education Abraham Flexner (1865–1959) was the first to develop an encompassing view on how clinical medicine should be taught. He distinguished three formats: (1) study or observation of the individual patient throughout the whole course of the disease by the student under proper guidance and control, (2) demonstration of cases by the instructor, and (3) the exposition of principles (Flexner 1925) (p. 238–239). Flexner strongly advocated bringing the student into close and active relation with the patient (Bonner 2002) (p. 84). Most importantly, he saw the teaching clinic as a laboratory, similar to that in the basic sciences, though lagging behind in scientific rigor (Ludmerer 1985). In his view, the scientific approach, which had been so successful to advance physiology, pathology, and biochemistry, could directly be transferred to the bedside: "There are no principles involved in teaching clinical medicine that are not likewise involved in the teaching of the laboratory subjects" (Flexner 1925) (p. 237). The thinking processes of clinicians proceeded along exactly the same lines as those of scientists, he claimed (Flexner 1925) (p. 10). Even the most brilliant demonstration, Flexner believed, was less educative than a "more or less bungled experiment" carried out by the student (Flexner 1912) (p. 84). The response of the medical community in Flexner's time was ambivalent: at a more abstract level, many physicians and teachers endorsed the view that diagnostic problem solving could benefit from a scientific approach (Becker et al. 1961) (p. 223); but at a more concrete level, they found Flexner's views unpalatable, as he rejected as unscientific many clinical practices that in their eyes were inevitable, such as "intelligent guesswork," the "tentative interpretation of fragmentary information," and what Flexner disparagingly described as "improvised therapy consisting of little more than persuasion sustained only by the physician's authority and personality" (Miller 1966) (p. 651). Unlike scientists, clinicians cannot indefinitely postpone their judgments and go on collecting further evidence that may enable them eventually to draw firm conclusions; hence, even though students can be trained to do scientific research, the scientific approach Flexner propagated cannot be directly applied to clinical problems.

Half a century later, it was clear that Flexner's recommendations for a more scientific approach to teaching clinical reasoning had not fallen in fertile soil. On the contrary, Becker et al. (1961) observed that teaching in the clinic was haphazard and consisted largely of residents teaching the students those things which are "closest to the students' hearts," namely, "procedure, "pearls," tips, and other bits of medical wisdom which the resident suspects will be useful for the practicing physician" (Becker et al. 1961) (p. 357). When a student asked a question, "which sounded perfectly reasonable," Becker et al. (1961) noted the supervisor-clinician frequently gave an answer that started with "In my experience…" and rarely came up with arguments that "carry the force of reason or logic" (Becker et al. 1961) (p. 235). In other words, arguments of persuasion, authority, and experience predominated in the clinic over a more reasoned and systematic approach. Though Becker et al.'s (1961) observations were limited to a single medical school, there is no evidence that the situation was different in other medical schools in the 1950s and 1960s. For example, in an extensive discussion of the new medical curriculum at Western Reserve University in the 1950s, clinical science is defined as "observing and working with patients" (Williams 1980) (p. 162), but no details about clinical problem solving are provided. The fact that Elstein et al. (1972) started their research project on medical problem solving with an exploratory study of how experienced physicians solve diagnostic problems illustrates the belief that little was known about how physicians actually solve clinical problems, let alone how they could teach this in a systematic fashion.

Early Diagnostic Tools, Computer-Assisted Instruction (CAI), and Patient Management Problems

If the art of clinical reasoning cannot be taught and the science of clinical reasoning cannot be applied, are there any options left for teaching clinical reasoning? In the 1950s, a third approach appeared on the stage: diagnosis as applied technology (Balla 1985) (p. 1). Two interrelated developments fueled this view: first, new mathematical and statistical techniques were applied to medical diagnosis; second, the development of the electronic computer opened a window to apply these mathematical and statistical, as well as other analytic, methods, to clinical problem solving. In 1954, Firmin Nash (at the time the director of the South West London Mass X-Ray Service) presented the "Logoscope," a device analogous to a slide rule, with removable columns which allowed the manipulation of any sample of qualitative clinical data (Nash 1954, 1960). The Logoscope embodied the concept of a disease manifestation matrix, a table with the columns representing disease, and the rows signs, symptoms, or laboratory findings (Jacquez 1964). The Logoscope was the first mechanistic tool to help the diagnostician focus on relevant diagnostic hypotheses, after collecting the (clinical) findings of a specific patient. In the 1960s, the first digital computer programs were written that aimed at instructing students how to solve clinical problems. Given the limited availability of computers and the highly constrained way humans could interact with them, these programs should be seen as experimental systems, rather than as real teaching tools. Clinicians and computer programmers cooperated to preconceive every possible step in the diagnostic process the problem solver (student) could take and the machine's response to each step. By using "branched programming," an illusion of flexibility could be created, that is, the student could ask questions and suggest actions or diagnoses by selecting them from a vocabulary list (the precursor of today's "menu") to which the computer could then provide appropriate, though "canned," responses. Some programs even enabled the teacher to program a "pedagogic strategy" to guide the student's problem-solving process (Feurzeig et al. 1964). Predictable erroneous solution paths could, at least in theory, be recognized, and more appropriate alternative actions could be proposed. A slightly more advanced version of this type of early computer-assisted instruction (CAI) was able to generate "cases" as well: given a particular diagnosis, it could select symptoms and other findings on a statistical basis to characterize the "patient" (McGuire 1963). As teaching instruments, however, these programs could only provide case-specific recommendations, and in this respect, their scope was limited to "diagnostic drill" (Feurzeig et al. 1964). That is, the instructions did not embody an explicit general method to solve clinical problems which could be applied across different cases.

Primarily developed for assessment purposes, but to a limited extent also applicable in teaching contexts, is the conceptually similar, but paper-and-pencil-based approach called "patient management problems" (McCarthy and Gonella 1967; McGuire 1963). The method aims at simulating an actual clinical situation representative of a physician's practice. Like the early CAI systems, PMPs use branched programming, i.e., the student or clinician can choose from a repertory of possible actions; once an action is chosen, feedback is provided about the outcome. In practice, the user has to erase an opaque overlay designating the chosen action, after which feedback (e.g., results of a laboratory test) becomes visible. PMPs can be used in a teaching context by adapting the feedback, e.g., by providing reasons why the action was inadequate or by referring to literature. In line with the, at the time predominant, behavioristic view of learning, the immediate availability of feedback – without a teacher being physically present – was considered an important asset of the method (McCarthy and Gonella 1967). As PMPs did not allow for (legitimate) flexibility in the way a user can approach a clinical problem, the method became into disuse.

Artificial Intelligence and Problem-Based Learning

Artificial intelligence (AI) is a computer program characterized by flexibility and adaptivity; they do not rely on preprogrammed cases and fixed problem-solving routes, but can accommodate a broad range of user input and react with a similarly broad range of responses, including feedback and recommendations about how to proceed. When applied to complex, knowledge-rich domains, such as medicine, AI programs are called expert systems, and in education, they are known as intelligent tutoring systems (ITS). The fundamentals of all these programs are the same: chains of simple operations (jointly called programs) applied to simple content (basically, arrays of alphanumeric symbols). Complex procedures and complex knowledge emerge by assembling large numbers of simple operations and applying these to large amounts of simple content. In clinical medicine, AI refers to automated diagnostic systems featured by a strict distinction between disease knowledge on the one hand and diagnostic procedures on the other (Clancey 1984). In the 1980s, the heydays of this form of AI, several diagnostic systems were developed, of which INTERNIST (Miller et al. 1982) and MYCIN (Clancey 1983) are the most well-known. GUIDON-MANAGE (Rodolitz and Clancey 1989) was specifically developed to introduce medical students to the process of diagnostic reasoning and is probably the most prominent example of an ITS in medical diagnosis.

In fact, AI heavily draws on principles of human problem solving that, in their turn, were derived from the features of early programmable machines developed in the decades before AI itself was technically possible (Feigenbaum and Feldman 1963; Newell and Simon 1972). In the 1960s, this approach to problem solving was already described at a theoretical level in several publications on clinical problem solving (Gorry and Barnett 1968; Kleinmuntz 1965, 1968; Overall and Williams 1961; Wortman 1972, 1966). From an educational perspective, this appeared a promising approach: if general methods or procedures to solve clinical problems can be formulated independently from clinical content knowledge (Jacquez 1964), the process of clinical diagnosis can be taught directly (Gorry 1970) and applied irrespective of the content of the specific problem. The educational approach directly connected with this view of problem solving in medicine is problem-based learning (PBL) (Barrows 1983; Barrows and Tamblyn 1980; Neufeld and Barrows 1974). In the educational philosophy of McMaster University Medical School in Hamilton, Canada – the cradle of problem-based learning – becoming a problem solver was an explicit goal of the medical curriculum, apart from the physician as content expert. Like Gorry (1970), Barrows (1983) believed that a problem-solving approach or problem-solving skills could be directly taught. In this respect, however, PBL has not lived up to its promises – today, the method is conceived in entirely different terms, i.e., as an instructional approach that aims to integrate basic science and clinical knowledge (Schmidt 1983, 1993), but with little direct benefit for teaching clinical reasoning. How did this come about? The belief that it would be possible to develop a clear-cut method to solve clinical and diagnostic problems was dealt a fatal blow by Elstein et al. (1978) who extensively investigated differences between experts' and novices' approaches to these problems. Experts and novices alike solve diagnostic problems by generating a small number of hypotheses early in the process and then proceed by collecting evidence to confirm (or refute) these hypotheses. The only difference is that experts on the average generate better, i.e., more promising, hypotheses early in the clinical encounter (Hobus et al. 1987; Neufeld et al. 1981). Experts' superior performance in clinical diagnosis seems to be an inherent consequence of the knowledge structures they develop over the years as a consequence of their experience. As Elstein observes, "there is not much that formal theories of problem solving, judgment and decision making can do to facilitate this slow process" (Elstein 1995) (p. 53–54). Elstein et al.'s (1978) additional finding of expertise being highly case specific suggests that exposing students to a broad range of clinical problems might be the only feasible approach to teach clinical reasoning.

After Medical Problem Solving (1978): A Role Left for Teaching Clinical Reasoning?

Today, many researchers and clinical educators distinguish between two approaches of clinical problem solving: one based on pattern recognition or "pure induction" and one that is usually referred to as "hypothesis generation and testing" (Gale 1982; Norman 2005; Patel et al. 1993). In fact, the former can be seen as a limiting case of the latter, that is, when a physician recognizes a clinical condition with sufficient confidence to immediately (probably unconsciously) suppress all alternative hypotheses that might crop up, without a need for further confirmation. Though praised as the "mainspring of diagnosis" by some, e.g. McCormick (1986), the ability to recognize a multitude of patterns requires extensive experience and is, unlike reasoning, not amenable to direct instruction (Elstein 1995). This leaves us with hypothesis generation and testing as the focus of a diagnostic problem-solving method (Barrows and Feltovich 1987). However, this is a very general approach that humans use to solve all kinds of problems; it lacks the necessary specificity to be applicable to concrete clinical cases (Blois 1984). Thus, alternative approaches have been formulated. For example, Blois claims that if a clinician does not recognize a pattern, he/she nearly always reverts to a causal inquiry, trying to relate specific findings to general physiological or pathological conditions (Blois 1984; Edwards et al. 2009) or to what Ploger (1988) calls "known pathology." As this form of causal reasoning almost always involves some uncertainty – some steps in the causal sequence are not observable, but have to be inferred – the solution of a diagnostic problem will always be a *differential diagnosis*, rather than *the* diagnosis. Several authors have expressed doubts whether students can be taught to construct differential diagnoses for clinical cases (Papa et al. 2007). According to Elstein (1995) and Kassirer and Kopelman (Kassirer et al. 2010), there even is no agreed-upon definition of a differential diagnosis. An alternative approach is to group individual findings that for some reason "belong together," e.g., appear to have the same cause or are part of a known syndrome. Eddy and Clanton (1982) developed an approach to diagnosis that starts with clustering elementary findings into "aggregate findings." Next, a differential diagnosis (list of possible causes) is constructed for the most important aggregate finding, which they call the "pivot." Then, all elementary findings in the case that cannot be subsumed under the pivot are checked against the alternatives in the differential diagnosis of the pivot. If all elementary findings are covered by the differential diagnosis of the pivot, this is the differential diagnosis for the entire case. If not, the process will be repeated with the second aggregate finding now becoming the pivot and so on. Finally, the alternative options (diagnoses) in the DD can be listed as more or less likely. Given the information available, this might be the best possible solution of the case. The advantage of the approach is that it will often be easier to construct a differential diagnosis for a selected collection of findings than for an entire case, in particular if the number of signs, symptoms, and findings is large.

Evans and Gadd present a similar, but slightly more hierarchical approach (Evans and Gadd 1989). They distinguish six levels, ranging from the "empirium" (raw, uninterpreted findings) to the "global complex" which covers not only the diagnosis but also prevention and medical, social, and psychological care. The equivalent of Eddy and Clanton's (1982) pivot is called "facet" by Evans and Gadd (1989). Facets are sub-diagnostic, complex clusters of findings which can be attributed to a coherent underlying pathophysiological process. "Anemia" would be a good example of a facet. Evans and Gadd (1989) put a stronger emphasis on pathophysiological thinking than Eddy and Clanton (1982), but they are less explicit about how to construct a differential diagnosis. A third method that resembles the previous two approaches is the clinical problem analysis (CPA) (Custers et al. 2000). This approach is based on Weed's (1968a, b) "problem-oriented medical record." The "patient problem" in CPA is similar to Eddy and Clanton's (1982) "pivot" and Evans and Gadd's (1989) "facet" but has a more practical nature: a "patient problem" can be anything in a case for which a differential diagnosis can be constructed or that may require treatment or further diagnostic action. A critical aspect of the method is that uncertainty is captured by the differential diagnosis, rather than by the patient problem (patient problems are always clear, specific, and certain). Thus, a patient problem can never include likelihood qualifiers, such as "probably X" or "suspicion of Y." If two findings cannot be subsumed by the same patient problem with certainty, they should be made separate patient problems that require individual analysis. In this approach, the pitfall of "premature closure" – the tendency to stop considering other options after generating a tentative early hypothesis (Graber et al. 2005) – can be avoided, though at the expense of "incomplete synthesis" (the diagnostician may fail to appropriately aggregate findings, and this may slow down the diagnostic process) (Voytovich et al. 1986). But, provided that slowing down is acceptable in the case of clinicians who are still in training, this approach can be used in an educational context.

Teaching Clinical Reasoning: A Few General Recommendations

Today, few medical educators believe that there exists a single clinical reasoning method that can be applied to all diagnostic problems by diagnosticians of all stripes. Yet, this does not imply that one cannot teach beyond "repeated practice [–] on a similar range of problems" (Elstein et al. 1978) or "observing others engaged in the process" (Kassirer and Kopelman 1991). What can be done? Our suggestion would be that if clinical reasoning can neither be taught as a "pure" process nor directly as a skill, teaching it in a case-based format might be a proper middle ground. What further features may an effective case-based approach require? First, it is important to take the term "reasoning" seriously. The teacher or supervisor should avoid to overly emphasize the outcome (the "correct" diagnosis), for this may reinforce undesirable behavior, such as guessing or jumping to conclusions. In addition, teaching should consist of small steps and teachers should not hesitate to frequently ask hypothetical questions or questions that probe a possible explanation of findings, such as "What if…?", "Can you think of other possibilities?", "Can you explain this?", etc. It should also be clear to the participants (teacher and students) that a differential diagnosis is a legitimate endpoint of the process, particularly if different (diagnostic or therapeutic) actions are associated with each alternative in the differential diagnosis. There is limited evidence that a model schema characterizing disease into eight groups (congenital, traumatic, immunologic, neoplastic, metabolic, infectious, toxic, and vascular) can be helpful (Brawer et al. 1988), but any other approach, as long as it is systematic, may also be used by beginning students (Fulop 1985). Moreover, to be effective, objectives and expectations must be clearly communicated before clinical reasoning session begins (Edwards et al. 2009). The best format appears to be a small group session guided by a clinical tutor; in advanced groups, students can be asked to prepare and present a case. During sessions, students should be encouraged to actively participate and take notes – the importance of which was already emphasized by William Osler. To avoid the "retrospective bias" – teaching problem solving as if one is working toward a solution known in advance – the method works best when the teacher or tutor is not familiar with the case but has access to exactly the same information as the students (Kassirer 2010; Kassirer and Kopelman 1991). Critics might argue that this is a reduced form of clinical problem solving – and it is, deliberately so – for clinical reasoning is demanding and involves a high cognitive load (Qiao et al. 2014; Young et al. 2014); hence, it cannot be properly taught in an authentic context, where students simultaneously have to deal with a real patient: in this context, dealing with a real patient would impose "extraneous load" to the detriment of the "germane load," i.e., learning (van Merriënboer and Sweller 2010). On the other hand, in clinical reasoning sessions, students will learn how to deal with a case report or case record, an aspect of clinical practice that is difficult to train in practical context. In sum, teaching clinical reasoning in a step-by-step fashion, with an emphasis on formulating a correct and comprehensive differential diagnosis, will be the best way to start clinical training of junior medical students.

References

Balla, J. (1985). *The diagnostic process. A model for clinical teachers.* Cambridge, UK: Cambridge University Press.
Barrows, H. S. (1983). Problem-based, self-directed learning. *JAMA: The Journal of the American Medical Association, 250*(22), 3077. http://doi.org/10.1001/jama.1983.03340220045031.
Barrows, H. S., & Feltovich, P. J. (1987). The clinical reasoning process. *Medical Education, 21*(2), 86–91. http://doi.org/10.1111/j.1365-2923.1987.tb00671.x.
Barrows, H. S., & Tamblyn, R. M. (1980). *Problem-based learning. An approach to medical education.* New York: Springer.

Becker, H., Geer, B., Huges, E., & Strauss, A. (1961). *Boys in white. Student culture in medical school*. Chicago: University of Chicago Press.

Blois, M. (1984). *Information and medicine: The nature of medical descriptions*. Berkeley: University of California Press.

Bonner, T. N. (2002). *Iconoclast. Abraham Flexner and a life in learning*. Baltimore: Johns Hopkins University Press.

Brawer, M., Witzke, D., Fuchs, M., & Fulginiti, J. (1988). A schema for teaching differential diagnosis. *Proceedings of the Annual Conference of Research in Medical Education, 27*, 162–166.

Bridenbaugh, C. (1947). Dr Thomas Bond's essay on the utility of clinical lectures. *Journal of the History of Medinice and the Allied Sciences, 2*(1), 10–19.

Clancey, W. J. (1983). The epistemology of a rule-based expert system—A framework for explanation. *Artificial Intelligence, 20*(3), 215–251. http://doi.org/10.1016/0004-3702(83)90008-5.

Clancey, W. (1984). Methodology for building an intelligent tutoring system. In W. Kintsch, J. Miller, & P. Polson (Eds.), *Method and tactics in cognitive science* (pp. 51–83). Hillsdale: Lawrence Erlbaum Associates.

Custers, E. J., Stuyt, P. M., & De Vries Robbé, P. F. (2000). Clinical problem analysis (CPA): A systematic approach to teaching complex medical problem solving. *Academic Medicine, 75*(3), 291–297.

Eddy, D., & Clanton, C. (1982). The art of diagnosis: Solving the clinicopathological exercise. *New England Journal of Medicine, 306*(21), 1263–1268.

Edwards, J. C., Brannan, J. R., Burgess, L., Plauche, W. C., & Marier, R. L. (2009). Case presentation format and clinical reasoning: A strategy for teaching medical students. *Medical Teacher, 9*, 285.

Elstein, A. (1995). Clinical reasoning in medicine. In J. Higgs & M. Jones (Eds.), *Clinical reasoning in the health professions* (pp. 49–59). Oxford: Butterworth Heinemann.

Elstein, A., Kagan, N., Shulman, L., Jason, H., & Loupe, M. (1972). Methods and theory in the study of medical inquiry. *Journal of Medical Education, 47*, 85–92.

Elstein, A. S., Shulman, L. S., & Sprafka, S. A. (1978). *Medical problem solving. An analysis of clinical reasoning*. Cambridge, MA: Harvard University Press.

Evans, D., & Gadd, C. (1989). Managing coherence and context in medical problem-solving discourse. In D. Evans & V. L. Patel (Eds.), *Cognitive science in medicine: biomedical modelling* (pp. 211–255). Cambridge, MA: The MIT press.

Feigenbaum, E., & Feldman, J. (1963). *Computers and thought: A collection of articles*. New York: McGraw-Hill.

Feurzeig, W., Munter, P., Swets, J., & Breen, M. (1964). Computer-aided teaching in medical diagnosis. *Journal of Medical Education, 39*(8), 746–754.

Flexner, A. (1910). Medical education in the United States and Canada. A report to the Carnegie Foundation for the Advancement of Teaching. In ForgottenBooks (Ed.)., 2012 Repr. Boston: D.B. Updike, the Merrymount Press.

Flexner, A. (1912). *Medical education in Europe. A report to the Carnegie Foundation for the Advancement of Teaching, Bulletin #6*. New York: USA: The Carnegie Foundation.

Flexner, A. (1925). *Medical education. A comparative study*. New York: The MacMillan Company.

Fulop, M. (1985). Teaching differential diagnosis to beginning clinical students. *The American Journal of Medicine, 79*(6), 745–749. http://doi.org/10.1016/0002-9343(85)90526-1.

Gale, J. (1982). Some cognitive components of the diagnostic thinking process. *British Journal of Psychology, 52*(1), 64–76.

Gorry, G. (1970). Modeling the diagnostic process. *Journal of Medical Education, 45*(5), 293–302.

Gorry, G. A., & Barnett, G. O. (1968). Experience with a model of sequential diagnosis. *Computers and Biomedical Research, 1*(5), 490–507. http://doi.org/10.1016/0010-4809(68)90016-5.

Graber, M. L., Franklin, N., & Gordon, R. (2005). Diagnostic error in internal medicine. *Archives of Internal Medicine, 165*(13), 1493–1499. http://doi.org/10.1001/archinte.165.13.1493.

Hobus, P. P. M., Schmidt, H. G., Boshuizen, H. P. A., & Patel, V. L. (1987). Contextual factors in the activation of first diagnostic hypotheses: Expert-novice differences. *Medical Education, 21*(6), 471–476. http://doi.org/10.1111/j.1365-2923.1987.tb01405.x.

Jacquez, J. (1964). The diagnostic process: Problems and perspectives. In J. Jacquez (Ed.), *The diagnostic process* (pp. 23–37). Ann Arbor: University of Michigan Medical School.

Kassirer, J. P. (2010). Teaching clinical reasoning: Case-based and coached. *Academic Medicine, 85*(7), 1118–1124.

Kassirer, J., & Kopelman, R. (1991). *Learning clinical reasoning*. Baltimore: Lippincott Williams & Wilkins.

Kleinmuntz, B. (1965). Diagnostic problem solving by computer. *Japanese Psychological Research, 7*(4), 189–194. http://doi.org/10.4992/psycholres1954.7.189.

Kleinmuntz, B. (1968). The processing of clinical information by man and machine. In B. Kleinmuntz (Ed.), *Formal representation of human judgment*. New York: Wiley.

Ludmerer, K. M. (1985). *Learning to heal. The development of American medical education*. New York: Basic Books.

Mangrulkar, R. S., Saint, S., Chu, S., & Tierney, L. M. (2002). What is the role of the clinical "pearl"? *The American Journal of Medicine, 113*(7), 617–624. http://doi.org/10.1016/S0002-9343(02)01353-0.

Maude, J. (2014). Differential diagnosis: The key to reducing diagnosis error, measuring diagnosis and a mechanism to reduce healthcare costs. *Diagnosis, 1*(1), 107–109. http://doi.org/10.1515/dx-2013-0009.

McCarthy, W. H., & Gonella, J. S. (1967). The simulated patient management problem: A technique for evaluating and teaching clinical competence. *British Journal of Medical Education, 1*(5), 348–352. http://doi.org/10.1111/j.1365-2923.1967.tb01730.x.

McCormick, J. (1986). Diagnosis: The need for demystification. *The Lancet, 328*(8521), 1434–1435.

McGuire, C. (1963). A process approach to the construction and analysis of medical examinations. *Journal of Medical Education, 38*, 556–563.

van Merriënboer, J. J. G., & Sweller, J. (2010). Cognitive load theory in health professional education: Design principles and strategies. *Medical Education, 44*(1), 85–93. http://doi.org/10.1111/j.1365-2923.2009.03498.x.

Miller, H. (1966). Fifty years after flexner. *The Lancet, 288*(7465), 647–654. http://doi.org/10.1016/S0140-6736(66)92827-3.

Miller, R., Pople, H., & Myers, J. (1982). INTERNIST-I, an experimental computer-based diagnostic consultant for general internal medicine. *New England Journal of Medicine, 307*(8), 468–476.

Nash, F. (1954). Differential diagnosis: An apparatus to assist the logical faculties. *Lancet, 263*(6817), 874–875.

Nash, F. (1960). Diagnostic reasoning and the logoscope. *Lancet, 276*(7166), 1442–1446.

Neufeld, V., & Barrows, H. (1974). The "McMaster philosophy": An approach to medical education. *Journal of Medical Education, 49*, 1040–1050.

Neufeld, V., Norman, G. R., Feighter, J. W., & Barrows, H. S. (1981). Clinical problem-solving by medical students: A cross-sectional and longitudinal analysis. *Medical Education, 15*(5), 315–322. http://doi.org/10.1111/j.1365-2923.1981.tb02495.x.

Newell, A., & Simon, H. (1972). *Human problem solving*. Englewood Cliffs: Prentice-Hall.

Norman, G. (2005). Research in clinical reasoning: Past history and current trends. *Medical Education, 39*(4), 418–427. http://doi.org/10.1111/j.1365-2929.2005.02127.x.

Overall, J. E., & Williams, C. M. (1961). Models for medical diagnosis. *Bahavioral Science, 6*(2), 134–141.

Papa, F. J., Oglesby, M. W., Aldrich, D. G., Schaller, F., & Cipher, D. J. (2007). Improving diagnostic capabilities of medical students via application of cognitive sciences-derived learning principles. *Medical Education, 41*(4), 419–425. http://doi.org/10.1111/j.1365-2929.2006.02693.x.

Patel, V. L., Groen, G. J., & Norman, G. R. (1993). Reasoning and instruction in medical curricula. *Cognition and Instruction, 10*(4), 335–378. http://doi.org/10.1207/s1532690xci1004_2.

Ploger, D. (1988). Reasoning and the structure of knowledge in biochemistry. *Instructional Science, 17*(1988), 57–76. http://doi.org/10.1007/BF00121234.

Qiao, Y.Q., Shen, J., Liang, X., Ding, S., Chen, F.Y., Shao, L., … Ran, Z.H. (2014). Using cognitive theory to facilitate medical education. *BMC Medical Education, 14*(1), 79. http://doi.org/10.1186/1472-6920-14-79.

Risse, G. (1989). Clinical instruction in hospitals: The Boerhaavian tradition in Leyden, Edinburgh, Vienna, and Padua. *Clio Medica, 21*, 1–19.

Rodolitz, N., & Clancey, W. (1989). GUIDON MANAGE: Teaching the process of medical diagnosis. In D. Evans & V. L. Patel (Eds.), *Cognitive science in medicine: Biomedical modeling* (pp. 313–348). Cambridge, MA: The MIT press.

Sanders, J. (2009). *Every patient tells a story. Medical mysteries and the art of diagnosis.* New York: Broadway Books. http://doi.org/10.1172/JCI41900.

Schmidt, H. (1983). Problem-based learning: Rationale and description. *Medical Education, 17*(1), 11–16.

Schmidt, H. G. (1993). Foundations of problem-based learning: Some explanatory notes. *Medical Education, 27*(5), 422–432. http://doi.org/10.1111/j.1365-2923.1993.tb00296.x.

Voytovich, A. E., Rippey, R. M., & Jue, D. (1986). Diagnostic reasoning in the multiproblem patient: An interactive, microcomputer-based audit. *Evaluation & the Health Professions, 9*(1), 90–102. http://doi.org/10.1177/016327878600900107.

Weed, L. (1968a). Medical records that guide and teach. *New England Journal of Medicine, 278*(12), 593–600.

Weed, L. (1968b). Medical records that guide and teach (concluded). *New England Journal of Medicine, 278*(12), 652–657.

Williams, G. (1980). *Western reserve's experiment on medical education and its outcome.* New York: Oxford University Press.

Wortman, P. M. P. (1966). Representation and strategy in diagnostic problem solving. *Human Factors, 8*(1), 48–53. http://doi.org/10.1177/001872086600800105.

Wortman, P. M. (1972). Medical diagnosis. An information processing approach. *Computers and Biomedical Research, 5*(4), 315–328.

Young, J. Q., Van Merrienboer, J., Durning, S., & ten Cate, O. (2014). Cognitive load theory: Implications for medical education: AMEE guide no. 86. *Medical Teacher, 36*(5), 371–384. http://doi.org/10.3109/0142159X.2014.889290.

Open Access This chapter is licensed under the terms of the Creative Commons Attribution 4.0 International License (http://creativecommons.org/licenses/by/4.0/), which permits use, sharing, adaptation, distribution and reproduction in any medium or format, as long as you give appropriate credit to the original author(s) and the source, provide a link to the Creative Commons license and indicate if changes were made.

The images or other third party material in this chapter are included in the chapter's Creative Commons license, unless indicated otherwise in a credit line to the material. If material is not included in the chapter's Creative Commons license and your intended use is not permitted by statutory regulation or exceeds the permitted use, you will need to obtain permission directly from the copyright holder.

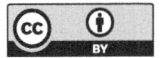

Chapter 3
Understanding Clinical Reasoning from Multiple Perspectives: A Conceptual and Theoretical Overview

Olle ten Cate and Steven J. Durning

Concepts and Definitions

This chapter is devoted to clarifying terminology and concepts that have been regularly cited and used in the last decades around clinical reasoning. Thus, this chapter represents a conceptual overview.

Success in clinical reasoning is essential to a physician's performance. Clinical reasoning is both a *process* and an *outcome* (with the latter often being referred to as decision-making). While these decisions must be evidence based as much as possible, clearly decisions also involve patient perspectives, the relationship between the physician and the patient, and the system or environment where care is rendered. Definitions of clinical reasoning therefore must include these aspects. While definitions of clinical reasoning vary, they typically share the features that clinical reasoning entails: (i) the cognitive operations allowing physicians to observe, collect, and analyze information and (ii) the resulting decisions for actions that take into account a patient's specific circumstances and preferences (Eva et al. 2007; Durning and Artino 2011).

The variety of definitions of clinical reasoning and the heterogeneity in research is likely in part due to the number of fields that have informed our understanding of clinical reasoning. In this chapter, a number of concepts from a broad spectrum of fields is presented to help the reader understand clinical reasoning and to assist the

---

O. ten Cate (✉)
Center for Research and Development of Education, University Medical Center Utrecht, Utrecht, The Netherlands
e-mail: T.J.tenCate@umcutrecht.nl

S.J. Durning
Uniformed Services University of the Health Sciences, Bethesda, MD, USA
e-mail: steven.durning@usuhs.edu

© The Author(s) 2018
O. ten Cate et al. (eds.), *Principles and Practice of Case-based Clinical Reasoning Education*, Innovation and Change in Professional Education 15,
https://doi.org/10.1007/978-3-319-64828-6_3

instruction of preclinical medical students. Many of these concepts reflect difficulties inherent to understanding how doctors think and how this type of thinking can be acquired by learners over time. Some provide hypotheses with more or less firm theoretical grounding, but a broad understanding of clinical reasoning requires an ongoing process of investigation.

Learning to Solve Problems in New Areas: Expanding the Learner Domain Space

Klahr and Dunbar proposed a model for scientific discovery (Klahr and Dunbar 1988) that may be helpful to understand how learners solve problems in unknown territory, such as what happens when a medical student starts learning to solve medical problems. The student has a *learner domain space* of knowledge that only partly overlaps, or not at all, with the *expert domain space* of knowledge, which is the space that contains all possible hypotheses a learner can generate about a problem. Knowledge building during inquiry learning can be considered as expanding the learner domain space to increase that overlap (Lazonder et al. 2008).

Early Thinking of Clinical Reasoning: The Computer Analogy

Building on the cognitive psychology work of Newell and Simon about problem-solving in the 1970s (Newell and Simon 1972), artificial intelligence (AI) computer models were created to resemble the clinical reasoning process, with programs like MYCIN and INTERNIST (Pauker et al. 1976). Analogies between cognitive functioning and the emerging computer capacities led to the assumption that both use algorithmic processes in the working memory, viewed as the *central processing unit* of the brain. Many predicted that like in chess, computer programs for medical diagnosis would quickly be developed and would perform superiorly to the practicing professional, outperforming the diagnostic accuracy of the best physician's thinking. Four decades later, however, this has not yet happened and may be impossible. The emergence of self-driving cars as an analogy shows how humans can build highly complex machines, but at least this development in clinical reasoning has been much slower than many had thought it would (Wachter 2015; Clancey 1983). Robert Wachter, in a recent book about technology in health care, argues that, still better than computers, experienced physicians can distinguish between patients with similar signs and symptoms to determine that "that guy is sick, and the other is okay," with the "the eyeball test" or intuition, which computers have not been able to capture so far (page 95), just as a computer cannot currently analyze nonverbal information that is so critical to communication in health care. Clinical decision support systems (CDSS, containing a large knowledge base and if-then rules for inferences) have been used with some success at the point of care to support clinicians in decision-making, particularly in medication decisions, but, integrated with electronic health records, they have not been shown to improve clinical outcome parameters as of yet (Moja et al. 2014).

Abandoning Clinical Reasoning as a General Problem-Solving Ability

Expertise in clinical reasoning was initially viewed as being synonymous with acquiring general problem-solving procedures (Newell and Simon 1972). However, in a groundbreaking study, published as a book in 1978 (*Medical Problem Solving*), Elstein and colleagues found few differences between expert (attending physicians) and novice diagnosticians (medical students) in the *way* they solve diagnostic problems (Elstein et al. 1978). The primary difference appeared to be in their knowledge and in particular the way it is structured as a consequence of experience. Thus while medical students and practicing physicians generated a similar number of diagnostic hypotheses differential diagnosis of similar length, practicing physicians were far more likely to list the correct diagnosis. This insight replaced the era that was marked by the belief that clinical reasoning could be measured as a distinct skill that would result in superior performance regardless of the specifics of a patient's presentation. Content knowledge was shown to be very important but still does not guarantee success in clinical reasoning. Variation in clinical performance is a product of the expert's integration of his or her knowledge of the signs and symptoms of disease with contextual factors in order to arrive at an adaptive solution.

Deconstructing the Reasoning Process

In an overview in 2005, Patel and colleagues summarize the process of clinical reasoning in four stages: abstraction, abduction, deduction, and induction (Patel et al. 2005).

Abstraction can be viewed as generalization from a finding to a conclusion (hemoglobin <12 gm/dl in an adult male is labeled as "anemia").

Abduction is a backward reasoning process to explain why this adult male should have anemia. "Abductive reasoning" was first coined as a term by logician C.S. Peirce in the nineteenth century to signify a common process when a surprising observation takes place that leads to a hypothesis ("The lawn is wet! Ergo, it has probably rained.") and is based on knowledge of possible causations and must be tested ("but it could also be the neighbor's sprinkler"). Abduction is considered to be a primary means of acquiring new ideas in clinical reasoning (Bolton 2015).

Deduction is the process of testing the hypothesis (e.g., of anemia) through confirmation by expected other diagnostic findings: *if* conditions X and Y are met, inference Z *must* be true.

Induction is the process of generalization from multiple cases and more applicable in research than in individual patient care: if multiple patients show similar signs and symptoms, general rules may be created to explain new cases.

Part of this process is *forward-driven reasoning* (hypothesis generation through data), and another part is *backward-driven reasoning* (hypothesis testing) (Patel et al. 2005).

Knowledge Representations to Support Reasoning

In a 1996 review, Custers and colleagues categorized the thinking about the way physician's cognition is organized around clinical knowledge in three alternative frameworks and provided critical notes (Custers et al. 1996). These mental representations could have the form of *prototypes*, *instances*, or *semantic networks*. All three of these models have assets and drawbacks in their explanatory power for clinical reasoning. The prototype framework or prototype theory assumes that multiple encounters with related diseases lead physicians to remember the common denominators, resulting in single prototypes in long-term memory. The instances framework assumes that physicians actually remember the individual instances of patient encounters without abstraction, and context-specific (situation specific) information may be part of these instances. The semantic network theory posits the existence of nodes of information units, connected with other nodes in the network. The strength of the network and its nodes depends on the intensity of its use. *Schemas* and *illness scripts* are medically meaningful interconnected nodes that can be strengthened and adapted based on clinical experience.

Prototyping and Semantic Qualifiers

Georges Bordage introduced the term *semantic qualifiers* referring to the use of abstract, often binary, terms to help sort through and organize (e.g., chunk) patient information. They are "useful adjectives" that represent an abstraction of the situational clinical findings (Chang et al. 1998). A commonly cited example of the use of semantic qualifiers is translating a patient who is presenting with knee swelling and pain into a presentation of acute monarticular arthritis. Note three semantic qualifiers – "acute," "monoarticular," and "arthritis." The reason why these qualifiers are important is that the structure of clinical knowledge in the clinician's mind is organized with such qualifiers, as claimed by Bordage. To enable recognition and linkage, the clinician must first translate what she hears and sees into such terminology (Bordage 1994). An assumption is that the clinician's memory contains *prototypes* of diseases (Bordage and Zacks 1984), generalizable representations that enable recognition. Bordage stresses how semantically rich discourses about patients are associated with greater diagnostic accuracy (Bordage 2007).

Illness Script Theory

Custers recently summarized scripts as high-level conceptual knowledge structures in long-term memory, representing general event sequences, in which the individual events are interconnected by temporal and often causal or hierarchical relationships ("usually diabetes type II occurs a older age, a overweight is associated; late symptoms might include vascular problems in the retina, in the lower limbs and in other places"). Scripts are activated as integral wholes in appropriate contexts that should contain relevant variables, including clinical findings in the patient. "Slots" in the reasoning process can be filled with information present in the actual situation, retrieved from memory, or inferred from the context (Custers 2015). Illness scripts, first introduced by Barrows and Feltovich, are believed to be chunks in long-term memory that contain three components, enabling conditions (past history and causes), fault (pathophysiology), and consequences (signs and symptoms) (Feltovics and Barrows 1984), and are elaborated further by Schmidt and Boshuizen (1993). Illness scripts are stored in long-term memory as units with temporal (i.e., sequential) components, as a film script of unfolding events, and patients are remembered as instances of a script. With experience, physicians build a larger repertoire of illness scripts and more elaborated scripts.

Illness scripts are shaped by experience and continually refined throughout one's clinical practice. When an experienced physician initially sees a patient, his or her verbal and nonverbal information is thought to immediately activate relevant illness scripts. This effortless, fast thinking, or nonanalytic process is referred to as *script activation*. In some cases, only one script is activated, and in these cases, one may arrive at the correct diagnosis (e.g., "type II diabetes mellitus"). In other cases, multiple scripts are activated, and then theory holds that we choose the most likely diagnosis by comparing and contrasting alternative illness scripts that were activated (through analytic or slow thinking). Early learners may not activate any scripts when they initially see a patient, and experts may activate one or several illness scripts.

Encapsulation of Knowledge and the Intermediate Effect

With increasing clinical information stored as illness scripts in the long-term memory of the physician, diagnostic reasoning should steadily become more accurate. However, studies have shown that more novice clinicians (e.g., those just out of training such as recent graduates from residency education) sometimes outperform physicians who have been in practice for some time (e.g., "experts") on the recall of details from clinical cases seen. This finding was coined by Schmidt and Boshuizen as the *intermediate effect* (Schmidt and Boshuizen 1993). While inexperienced clinicians may consciously use pathophysiological thinking when solving clinical problems, the frequent use of similar thinking pathways leads to efficient shortcuts, and after a while it may no longer be possible to unfold these pathways. The pathophysiological knowledge about the disease becomes *encapsulated* into diagnostic labels or high-level simplified causal models that explain signs and symptoms (Schmidt and Mamede 2015).

System 1 and 2 Thinking as Dual Processes

Dual process theory refers to two processes that are thought to apply during reasoning (Croskerry et al. 2014). Briefly, dual process theory argues that we have two general thought processes. Fast thinking (sometimes called System I thinking or "nonanalytic" reasoning) is believed to be quick, subconscious, and typically effortless. An example of a fast thinking strategy is pattern recognition (Eva 2005). An example of pattern recognition in medicine would happen when a physician examines a patient with palpitations and immediately recognizes the cardinal features or "pattern" of Graves' disease, when also observing exophthalmia, fine resting tremor, and thyromegaly. Slow or analytic thinking (System 2 thinking) on the other hand is effortful and conscious. An example of System 2 thinking would be working through a patient's acid base status (e.g., calculating an anion gap, using Winter's formula, and calculating a delta-delta gap). Dual process theory has recently been popularized in the book *Thinking, Fast and Slow* by Daniel Kahneman (2011). More recent work with dual process theory argues that both of these processes are used simultaneously, e.g., it's not one or the other but rather one uses a combination of both fast and slow thinking in practice. In other words, fast and slow thinking can be viewed as a continuum (Custers 2013). Efficient clinical work requires fast thinking. The capacity of the working memory would be overloaded if analytic reasoning were required for all decisions in patient care (Young et al. 2014).

Case Specificity and Context Specificity

In Elstein and colleagues' seminal work on medical problem-solving (Elstein et al. 1978), researchers noted that physician performance on one patient or case did not predict performance on a subsequent content area or case, giving rise to the phenomenon of *case specificity*. These findings would be quite surprising if medical problem-solving were a general skill.

A second vexing problem in practice is the more recently highlighted phenomenon of *context specificity*. Context specificity refers to the finding that a physician can see two patients with the same chief complaint and the same (or nearly identical) symptoms and physical findings and have the same diagnosis, yet, in different contexts, arrive at different diagnoses (Durning et al. 2011). The context can be helpful to arrive at the correct diagnosis (Hobus et al. 1987) or harmful and lead to error (Eva 2005). In other words, something other than the "essential content" is driving the physician's clinical reasoning. Durning and Artino hold that the outcome of clinical reasoning is driven by the context, which includes the physician, the patient, the system, and their interactions (Durning and Artino 2011). The notion of system includes appointment length, appointment location, support systems, and clinic staffing (Durning and Artino 2011) and stresses the importance of the situation. One example of "situativity" is *situated cognition*, which breaks down an activity like clinical reasoning into physician, patient, and environment as well as interactions between these components. Clinical reasoning is believed to emerge from these factors and their interactions. Another example of situativity, *situated learning*, stresses participation in an activity and identity formation as learning versus the acquisition of generalized facts.

Clinical Reasoning and the Development of Expert Performance

Despite the finding that clinical reasoning is *content*-dependent and *context*-dependent, expertise in diagnostic and therapeutic reasoning in general varies among physicians even with similar experience. Some internists are considered better diagnosticians and some surgeons better operators that others. It remains useful to think of what leads to superb performance, as education can be a part of it (Asch et al. 2014). Indeed, many scholars prefer the term expert performance as opposed to expertise when referring to clinical reasoning as the former acknowledges the many nuances to this ability that we have outlined in this chapter.

For procedural performance, repetitive practice is key. Competence in colonoscopy requires experience with 150–200 colonoscopies under supervision (Ekkelenkamp et al. 2016). That competence improves with practice is not surprising and known from, for instance, in chess (De Groot 1978). Anecdotally, in the

1960s the Hungarian educational psychologist László Polgár was determined to raise his yet unborn children to become highly skilled in a specific domain and chose chess. All three daughters received careful, highly intensive training, from very young age on, and have become world-top chess players, two of which are currently considered the world's best female chess players. Psychologist Ericsson has generalized the idea that, rather than innate talent, *deliberate practice* is key to expert performance (Ericsson et al. 1993). He distinguishes three subsequent mental representations: a planning phase with clear performance goals, a translation to execution, and a representation for monitoring how well one does. Applications in medical training have been described (Ericsson 2015) but have mainly focused on procedures. Clinical reasoning may benefit from deliberate practice, and the work of Mamede et al., using deliberate practice, shows how reasoning can benefit as well (Mamede et al. 2014).

Reflection During Diagnostic Thinking

Donald Schön coined the terminology of *reflection in action* and *reflection on action*, as a description of thinking of high-level professionals (Schön 1983). Knowing what to do when you do it may not require much effort if actions are routine, but professionals with nonroutine tasks may often face small problems or questions that require instant adaptive action. Schön maintains that reflection-in-action must be practiced by learners becoming professionals. Mamede and colleagues developed the method of "structured reflection" to improve students' diagnostic reasoning (Mamede et al. 2010, 2014a, b). Structured reflection in the context of clinical reasoning means that problem-solvers explicitly match a patient's presentation (case) against every diagnosis they consider for that case. Mamede et al. demonstrated a beneficial effect of this approach. Detailed comparison of a patient's signs and symptoms with the already available and activated illness scripts and noticing similarities and discrepancies appears to be the mechanism behind this restructuring of knowledge as a consequence of structured reflection. The authors recommend deliberate reflection as a tool for learning clinical reasoning (Schmidt and Mamede 2015).

Bias and Error in Clinical Reasoning

The quality of clinical reasoning is often expressed in how few errors a physician makes. Some errors are typical enough to receive a label and stem from various sources of bias. In 2003 Kempainen et al. published a helpful overview of typical biases that happen in clinical reasoning and that should be attended to in education, which include the following (Kempainen et al. 2003):

Availability bias. A differential diagnosis is influenced by what is easily recalled, creating a false sense of prevalence.
Representative bias (or judging by similarity). Clinical suspicion is influenced solely by signs and symptoms and neglects prevalence of competing diagnoses.
Confirmation bias (or pseudodiagnosticity). Additional testing confirms suspected diagnosis but fails to test competing hypotheses.
Anchoring bias. Inadequate adjustment of a differential diagnosis in light of new data resulting in a final diagnosis unduly influenced by the starting point.
Bounded rationality bias (or search satisficing). Clinicians stop searching for additional diagnoses after the anticipated diagnosis is made leading to a *premature closure* of the reasoning process.
Outcome bias. A clinical decision is judged on the outcome rather than on the logic and evidence supporting the decision.

A limitation of this approach is that when the reasoning is believed to be successful, biases are not typically recognized, and when looking at a case in hindsight, many mistakes can easily be labeled as caused by "bias." Indeed, so-called biases actually may serve as heuristics to guide successful behavior (Gigerenzer and Gaissmaier 2011; Gigerenzer 2007). In a recent overview, Norman and colleagues conclude that interventions directed at error reduction through the identification of heuristics and biases have no effect on diagnostic errors. Instead, most errors seem to originate from a limited knowledge based of the clinician (Norman et al. 2017).

Neuroscience and Visual Expertise in Clinical Reasoning

While neuroscience is quickly uncovering many cognitive processes, clinical reasoning has hardly been subject of such studies. More recently however a new line of research has evolved which seeks to explore the biologic underpinnings of clinical reasoning. Indeed, an Achilles heel of clinical reasoning is that it is less subject to introspection or visualization, and thus these new methods such as functional magnetic resonance imaging (fMRI) and electroencephalogram (EEG) are emerging and show particular promise for enhancing our understanding of System 1 thinking. One of the first publications in this domain is from Durning et al. who studied brain process with functional MRI techniques in novices and experts solving clinical problems through vignette-based multiple choice questions. Many parts of the brain were activated. The researchers observed activity in various regions of the prefrontal cortex (Durning et al. 2015). While preliminary, fMRI may be a promising route of future investigation.

A new and related avenue of investigation is that of visual expertise (Bezemer 2017; van der Gijp et al. 2016). Medicine is a highly visual profession, not only for specific disciplines such as radiology, pathology, dermatology, surgery, and cardiology but also in primary care (Kok and Jarodzka 2017). Visually observing a patient, human tissue, or a representation of it, and recognizing abnormality, may not easily be expressed in words but can instantly lead to a System 1 recognition.

In Sum

The intention of this chapter was to provide an overview of theoretical concepts, frequently used terms, and a number of significant thinkers and authors in this domain, all of which underlie our current understanding of clinical reasoning to support the teaching of students about clinical reasoning in the preclinical period and beyond.

While much of the cited literature appeared after the model of case-based clinical reasoning was first created in 1992 (ten Cate 1994), and some aspects apply to clinical rather than preclinical education, none of the recommendations that could be drawn for this chapter would conflict the CBCR approach.

Although it is apparent that there are still numerous gaps in our collective understanding of clinical reasoning, it is also clear that progress into a more thorough understanding of clinical reasoning is advancing.

References

Asch, D. A., et al. (2014). How do you deliver a good obstetrician? Outcome-based evaluation of medical education. *Academic Medicine, 89*(1), 24–26.
Bezemer, J. (2017). Visual research in clinical education. *Medical Education, 51*(1), 105–113.
Bolton, J. W. (2015). Varieties of clinical reasoning. *Journal of Evaluation in Clinical Practice, 21,* n/a–n/a. Available at: http://doi.wiley.com/10.1111/jep.12309
Bordage, G. (1994). Elaborated knowledge: A key to successful diagnostic thinking. *Academic Medicine, 69*(11), 883–885.
Bordage, G. (2007). Prototypes and semantic qualifiers: From past to present. *Medical Education, 41*(12), 1117–1121.
Bordage, G., & Zacks, R. (1984). The structure of medical knowledge in the memories of medical students and general practitioners: Categories and prototypes. *Medical Education, 18*(11), 406–416.
Chang, R., Bordage, G., & Connell, K. (1998). The importance of early problem representation during case presentations. *Academic Emergency Medicine: Official Journal of the Society for Academic Emergency Medicine, 73*(10), S109–S111.
Clancey, W. J. (1983). The epistemology of a rule-based expert system – A framework for explanation. *Artificial Intelligence, 20*(3), 215–251.
Croskerry, P., et al. (2014). Deciding about fast and slow decisions. *Academic Medicine, 89*(2), 197–200.
Custers, E. J. F. M. (2013). Medical education and cognitive continuum theory: An alternative perspective on medical problem solving and clinical reasoning. *Academic Medicine, 88*(8), 1074–1080.
Custers, E. J. F. M. (2015). Thirty years of illness scripts: Theoretical origins and practical applications. *Medical Teacher, 37*(5), 457–462.
Custers, E., Regehr, G., & Norman, G. (1996). Mental representations of medical diagnostic knowledge: A review. *Academic Medicine, 71*(10), S55–S61.
De Groot, A. (1978). *Thought and choice in chess.* The Hague: Mouton.
Durning, S. J., & Artino, A. R. (2011). Situativity theory: A perspective on how participants and the environment can interact: AMEE guide no. 52. *Medical Teacher, 33*(3), 188–199.

Durning, S., et al. (2011). Context and clinical reasoning: Understanding the perspective of the expert's voice. *Medical Education, 45*(9), 927–938.

Durning, S. J., et al. (2015). Neural basis of nonanalytical reasoning expertise during clinical evaluation. *Brain and Behaviour, 309*, 1–10.

Ekkelenkamp, V. E., et al. (2016). Training and competence assessment in GI endoscopy: A systematic review. *Gut, 65*(4), 607–615. Available at: http://gut.bmj.com/content/65/4/607.abstract

Elstein, A. S., Shulman, L. S., & Sprafka, S. A. (1978). Medical problem solving. In *An analysis of clinical reasoning*. Cambridge, MA: Harvard University Press.

Ericsson, K. A. (2015). Acquisition and maintenance of medical expertise. *Academic Medicine, 90*(11), 1–16.

Ericsson, K. A., et al. (1993). The role of deliberate practice in the acquisition of expert performance. *Psychological Review, 100*(3), 363–406.

Eva, K. W. (2005). What every teacher needs to know about clinical reasoning. *Medical Education, 39*(1), 98–106.

Eva, K. W., et al. (2007). Teaching from the clinical reasoning literature: Combined reasoning strategies help novice diagnosticians overcome misleading information. *Medical Education, 41*(12), 1152–1158.

Feltovics, P. & Barrows, H. (1984). Issues of generality in medical problem solving. In H. Schmidt & M. De Volder (Eds), *Tutorials in problem-based learning* (pp. 128–142). Assen/Maastricht: Van Gorcum.

Gigerenzer, G. (2007). *Gut feelings. The intelligence of the unconscious*. New York: Penguin Group.

Gigerenzer, G., & Gaissmaier, W. (2011). Heuristic decision making. *Annual Review of Psychology, 62*, 451–482.

Hobus, P. P. M., et al. (1987). Contextual factors in the activation of first diagnostic hypotheses: Expert-novice differences. *Medical Education, 21*(6), 471–476.

Kahneman, D. (2011). *Thinking, fast and slow*. New York: Farrar, Straus and Giroux.

Kempainen, R. R., Migeon, M. B., & Wolf, F. M. (2003). Understanding our mistakes: A primer on errors in clinical reasoning. *Medical Teacher, 25*(2), 177–181.

Klahr, D., & Dunbar, K. (1988). Dual space search during scientific reasoning. *Cognitive Science, 12*(1), 1–48.

Kok, E. M., & Jarodzka, H. (2017). Before your very eyes: The value and limitations of eye tracking in medical education. *Medical Education, 51*(1), 114–122.

Lazonder, A. W., Wilhelm, P., & Hagemans, M. G. (2008). The influence of domain knowledge on strategy use during simulation-based inquiry learning. *Learning and Instruction, 18*(6), 580–592.

Mamede, S., et al. (2010). Effect of availability bias and reflective reasoning on diagnostic accuracy among internal medicine residents. *JAMA: The Journal of the American Medical Association, 304*(11), 1198–1203.

Mamede, S., van Gog, T., Sampaio, A. M., et al. (2014a). How can students' diagnostic competence benefit most from practice with clinical cases? The effects of structured reflection on future diagnosis of the same and novel diseases. *Academic Medicine: Journal of the Association of American Medical Colleges, 89*(1), 121–127.

Mamede, S., van Gog, T., van den Berge, K., et al. (2014b). Why do doctors make mistakes? A study of the role of salient distracting clinical features. *Academic Medicine: Journal of the Association of American Medical Colleges, 89*(1), 114–120.

Miller, G. A. (1956). The magical number seven, plus or minus two: Some limits on our capacity for processing information. *Psychological Review, 63*, 81–97.

Moja, L., et al. (2014). Effectiveness of computerized decision support systems linked to electronic health records: A systematic review and meta-analysis. *American Journal of Public Health, 104*(12), e12–e22.

Newell, A., & Simon, H. (1972). *Human problem solving*. Englewood Cliffs: Prentice-Hall.

Norman, G. R., et al. (2017). The causes of errors in clinical reasoning: Cognitive biases, knowledge deficits, and dual process thinking. *Academic Medicine, 92*(1), 23–30.

Patel, V., Arocha, J., & Zhang, J. (2005). Thinking and reasoning in medicine. In K. Holyoak & R. Morrison (Eds.), *The Cambridge handbook of thinking and reasoning* (pp. 727–750). Cambridge: Cambridge University Press.

Pauker, S., et al. (1976). Towards the simulation of clinical cognition: Taking the present illness by computer. *Americal Journal of Medicine, 60*, 981–996.

Schmidt, H. G., & Boshuizen, H. P. A. (1993). On acquiring expertise in medicine. *Educational Psychology Review, 5*(3), 205–221.

Schmidt, H. G., & Mamede, S. (2015). How to improve the teaching of clinical reasoning: A narrative review and a proposal. *Medical Education, 49*(10), 961–973.

Schön, D. A. (1983). *The reflective practitioner - how professionals think in action*. New York: Basic Books.

ten Cate, O. (1994). Training case-based clinical reasoning in small groups [Dutch]. *Nederlands Tijdschrift voor Geneeskunde, 138*, 1238–1243.

van der Gijp, A. et al. (2016). How visual search relates to visual diagnostic performance: A narrative systematic review of eye-tracking research in radiology. *Advances in Health Sciences Education*, 1–23.

Wachter, R. (2015). *The digital doctor – hope, hype, harm at the Dawn of medicine's computer age*. New York: McGraw-Hill.

Young, J. Q., et al. (2014). Cognitive load theory: Implications for medical education: AMEE guide no. 86. *Medical Teacher, 36*(5), 371–384.

Open Access This chapter is licensed under the terms of the Creative Commons Attribution 4.0 International License (http://creativecommons.org/licenses/by/4.0/), which permits use, sharing, adaptation, distribution and reproduction in any medium or format, as long as you give appropriate credit to the original author(s) and the source, provide a link to the Creative Commons license and indicate if changes were made.

The images or other third party material in this chapter are included in the chapter's Creative Commons license, unless indicated otherwise in a credit line to the material. If material is not included in the chapter's Creative Commons license and your intended use is not permitted by statutory regulation or exceeds the permitted use, you will need to obtain permission directly from the copyright holder.

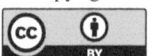

Chapter 4
Prerequisites for Learning Clinical Reasoning

Judith L. Bowen and Olle ten Cate

Introduction

To complement the elaboration of the specific method of case-based clinical reasoning (CBCR), this chapter is devoted to general competencies or prerequisites for clinical reasoning that may be acquired in parallel with the acquisition of illness script knowledge from the CBCR method.

Many medical schools design curricula and courses separating preclinical from clinical years, although that tradition has been challenged (Cooke et al. 2010). The designation "preclinical" connotes a curricular responsibility to prepare students for clinical experiences. Developing skills for clinical reasoning is an essential part of a larger, integrated identity that students will need to bring to clinical experiences in order to participate in caring for patients and work in teams. Communication skills are necessary for building rapport with patients, conducting the medical interview, engaging in shared decision-making with patients, eliciting patients' concerns and expectations, discussing clinical cases with colleagues and clinical supervisors, and explaining one's reasoning to others. Aper and colleagues have recently called this "complex competence" (Aper et al. 2014).

Effective clinical reasoning is one of the many competencies students must learn to master. So what can teachers do to promote students' readiness for clinical reasoning before patient care becomes their primary learning activity? In this chapter,

---

J.L. Bowen (✉)
Division of General Internal Medicine and Geriatrics, Oregon Health & Science University, Portland, OR, USA
e-mail: bowenj@ohsu.edu

O. ten Cate
Center for Research and Development of Education, University Medical Center Utrecht, Utrecht, The Netherlands
e-mail: T.J.tenCate@umcutrecht.nl

© The Author(s) 2018
O. ten Cate et al. (eds.), *Principles and Practice of Case-based Clinical Reasoning Education*, Innovation and Change in Professional Education 15, https://doi.org/10.1007/978-3-319-64828-6_4

we will briefly review the traditional educational approaches used to prepare students for immersive clinical experiences and then describe a set of sequential teaching strategies one might consider prerequisites for clinical reasoning. This proposed sequence includes *learning to talk like a physician*, i.e., using the clinical vocabulary; *identifying the clinical problem* to be solved, often called problem representation; *organizing case information* and schema development, i.e., building one's illness script mental repository; comparing and contrasting diagnostic hypotheses, which we will call *contrastive learning*; *identifying discriminating information* for hypothesis-driven inquiry; and *diagnostic verification* to enrich one's mental repository for use in clinical reasoning.

Preparing students to act in clinical rotations and to become involved with clinical reasoning and decision-making in practice is done in medical schools in very different ways, varying from virtually no practice with clinical reasoning to extensive training in lecture settings or small groups, using real or standardized patients, or with written or electronic cases. Traditionally, most medical schools require students to participate in introductory courses designed to teach clinical skills, such as communicating with patients, the medical interview, the physical examination, and clinical reasoning. Some of these courses are described in the literature (LaRochelle et al. 2009). The most common approach involves a longitudinal series of small groups using problem-based learning methods and simulated clinical cases (paper, electronic, or video recorded) or standardized patients to introduce clinical skill or reasoning content and provide opportunity for practice and discussion (Barrows and Tamblyn 1980). More recently, web-based learning and virtual patient encounters by simulation have been introduced to supplement small group experiences (Cook et al. 2010; Kim and Kee 2012). Another common approach is "transition to clerkship" courses designed as an intensive immersion experience for students just prior to beginning their first clerkship (Jacobson et al. 2010; O'Brien and Poncelet 2010). Common content areas include preparation for participation in clinical activities (including clinical reasoning), roles and expectations of students, advice from senior students, professionalism, stress management, and procedural skills.

Underlying any specific model of teaching and often quite implicit is the general purpose of the preparation for clinical reasoning in practice. The six components of this purpose outlined above constitute a general framework that may be addressed in any form of preparatory education. To be able to adequately contribute to the reasoning process of clinical teams, students must be prepared with a *clinical vocabulary*, with the ability to create clinical *problem representations*, with a foundational *illness script mental library*, and with habits of *contrastive learning*, *hypothesis-driven inquiry*, and *diagnostic verification*.

Clinical Vocabulary

Along with learning to think like a physician, medical students learn to talk like physicians. As with all knowledge communities, language is a defining element. The knowledge community of medicine is no exception. The best example of this phenomenon is the admonition to teach students to converse with patients in lay language familiar to the patient and "avoid medical jargon." Yet, when physicians talk together while trying to make sense of a clinical problem or determine the correct diagnosis, they do so using language specific to the practice of medicine. Why is this? There are several reasons why physicians among themselves must use medical terminology. First, numerous medical concepts, be they morphological structures, biochemical or physiological processes, disease entities, procedures of investigation, or medications, simply have no efficient non-jargon wordings ("acromion," "pernicious anemia," "osmosis," "Weber and Rinne hearing tests"). Next, verbal labels are powerful for summarizing combinations of features that would otherwise require extensive explanation ("toxic shock," "Cushing's syndrome"). Finally, medical vocabulary serves the uniformity of information exchange among professionals. While patients may express similar complaints in many different ways, medical terminology serves this uniformity. The outside world may sometimes view this communication among medical professionals as mysterious, ritualized, deliberately secretive to protect the profession as a closed community, and unnecessary, but the truth is that medical vocabulary is indispensible for efficient communication and safe care. Students simply must get acquainted with it.

Preclinical education introduces and reinforces language used to describe core science concepts in order to develop a shared understanding of the pathophysiological basis of disease. Similarly, learning the meaning of words that physicians assign to patients' stories of their illnesses is a prerequisite for learning clinical reasoning. Why is this important? By analyzing transcripts from medical students' and experienced physicians' oral case presentations, Bordage and colleagues have shown that the "think-aloud" discourse patterns of clinicians who eventually arrived at the correct diagnosis used language structures representative of a broad and deep understanding of the clinical problem (Bordage et al. 1997; Bordage and Lemieux 1991). Specifically, those physicians with greater diagnostic competence translated specific clinical features into abstract semantic qualifiers, which facilitated their ability to abstractly define the clinical problem that needed to be solved. Semantic qualifiers are adjectives or adverbs that represent an abstraction of the situational clinical findings (Chang et al. 1998). Examples of semantic qualifiers are shown in the third column of Tables 4.1 and 4.2. One small study among third-year medical students completing standardized patient examinations noted that students who used semantic qualifiers during case presentations as compared to those who simply reported the patient's signs and symptoms demonstrated stronger diagnostic competence (Bordage et al. 1997).

Importantly, training students to use semantic qualifiers in describing the patient's chief complaint and history of present illness is likely to improve their recollection of findings at a later moment, but not necessarily the accuracy of reasoning. Nendaz and Bordage were able to show that second-year medical students could learn to use semantic qualifiers to describe case features. The use of semantic qualifiers was associated with better case information recall but not with better diagnostic accuracy (Nendaz and Bordage 2002). Thus, learning how to talk like physicians should be viewed as a prerequisite condition for developing diagnostic reasoning competence, which in itself requires more. Teachers can encourage preclinical students to begin learning and using the vocabulary of such a semantically driven discourse.

Using a clinical example to illustrate the translation of a patient's story from lay language to semantic qualifiers, consider the following brief clinical history as conveyed by the patient:

> Alicia A. is a 55 year old woman who for the past 2 months has had stiffness of her hands on awakening each morning that lasts for 1–2 hours. She has felt weak and fatigued on several occasions. She has noticed swelling of both wrists and pain when attempting to make a fist. At first, the stiffness didn't bother her. Now, as a basic scientist with an active experimental laboratory, she is having difficulty using micro-pipettes to create her cell cultures.

Alicia becomes "female"; 55-year-old becomes "middle aged"; 2 months becomes "chronic"; stiffness on awakening each morning that lasts for 1–2 h becomes "morning stiffness" (as specifically defined and diagnostically meaningful in the field of rheumatology); weak and fatigued on several occasions become "recurrent, systemic"; both wrists become symmetrical small joints; and difficulty using micro-pipettes becomes "moderately severe." Translated using semantic qualifiers, the story becomes:

> A middle aged female presents with a chronic, recurrent, moderately severe systemic illness characterized by fatigue and morning stiffness in bilateral, symmetrical small joints of the hands.

When introducing new clinical cases for students' consideration, teachers can write the patient's history using common or "lay" language descriptions, similar to the way patients most often portray their stories, and then ask students to translate the case findings into abstract terms. Further, students' review of these clinical histories related to the patient's reason for the visit can be structured to assure thoroughness (Hasnain et al. 2001). A clear focus on and thoroughness of inquiry about the chief complaint early in the patient interview has been associated with stronger diagnostic competence (Hasnain et al. 2001). To encourage students to form strong habits for thorough exploration of the chief complaint, preclinical students may benefit from practice in building their clinical vocabulary with a structured format focused on the basic semantic attributes of the reason for visit and history of present illness: onset, site or location, severity, course or chronology, context including setting and patient characteristics, and aggravating or alleviating factors (Chang et al. 1998; Nendaz and Bordage 2002; Skeff 2014). Table 4.1 shows how a patient's history, described using lay terms, is translated to the medical vocabulary.

In some cases, the abstract translation may be obvious, and, through discussion, students will reach consensus quickly, with or without guidance. In other instances,

Table 4.1 Translation of a patient's history using semantic qualifiers (A)

Structured inquiry of reason for visit	Patient's story described using lay terms	Abstract translation using semantic qualifiers
Symptom onset	"At first the stiffness didn't bother"	Gradual, progressive
Symptom site/location	"Stiffness of her hands"	Small joints, symmetrical
Symptom severity	"Stiffness on awakening lasting 1–2 h," "difficulty using micro-pipettes"	Moderate to severe morning stiffness
Symptom course/chronology	"2 months"	Chronic
Context/patient characteristics	"55-year-old," "Alicia"	Middle-aged female

the meaning assigned to abstract vocabulary terms will come with greater experience and may be context specific. For example, when does an acute problem become subacute or chronic? When does an oligoarticular problem become polyarticular? Students will need to learn the importance of clarifying the meaning of specific words when discussing clinical cases to facilitate a shared understanding of the clinical problem.

Clinical cases illustrating limb or joint problems lend themselves nicely to learning the meaning of proximal versus distal, symmetrical versus asymmetrical, axial versus appendicular, and mono- versus oligo- versus polyarticular joint complaints. Other clinical presentations, such as those of many cardiovascular, renal, or neurological problems, are typically general or systemic in nature and defining the symptom site is more difficult. Students should be encouraged to recognize and name symptoms of a systemic nature such as fatigue, malaise, or confusion.

A second clinical case illustrates this difference:

> Robert is a 28 year old male brought by his friends to the emergency room after he collapsed during the initial part of his first soccer match. His friends report loss of consciousness of about 30 seconds. Robert reports difficulty breathing, especially when lying down. He has experienced mild shortness of breath when exercising ever since he can remember, but his symptoms now are a lot worse. In retrospect, his exercise tolerance has been declining for the past 9–12 months. He used to be able to do almost anything he wanted but now notices that he gets quite breathless after only a flight of stairs. On two occasions about 4 months ago he had to stop walking up stairs because of chest pain, which scared him. He describes the chest pain as tightness in the middle of his chest that never lasts longer than a minute and goes away with rest.

Table 4.2 illustrates the semantic transformation for this case. Using a similarly explicit approach, Skeff emphasizes the *chronology* of the present illness as a way of making sense out of a complex history of present illness. In this approach, *time* is the core structural element ("overtly identifying times when symptoms appeared or changed"). Advantages of this approach include attending to subtle or puzzling changes in the presentation and finding clues to the pathophysiological process, neither ignoring nor overemphasizing specific symptoms (Skeff 2014).

Table 4.2 Translation of a patient's history using semantic qualifiers (B)

Structured inquiry of reason for visit	Patient's story	Abstract translation using semantic qualifiers
Symptom onset	"He collapsed," "about 30 seconds," "chest tightness, never longer than a minute"	Sudden
		Episodic
Symptom site/location	"Loss of consciousness"	Systemic or constitutional
	"Difficulty breathing"	Respiratory/cardiovascular
Symptom severity	"(Declining) exercise tolerance" "quite breathless after a flight of stairs"	Moderate to severe
Symptom course/chronology	"Declining for the past 9–12 months," "used to be able to do almost anything he wanted"	Chronic, progressive
Context/patient characteristics	"28-year-old," "Robert"	Young male
Aggravating/alleviating factors	"Goes away with rest"	Resolves

Problem Representation

Once students have started to learn the vocabulary physicians use to describe patients' clinical concerns, they will be ready to begin using these words to formulate the clinical problem that the case requires them to solve. This clinical problem formulation is called the problem representation. A problem representation combines the situational information about the patient with the clinician's knowledge to create a structured and actionable description of the problem (Feltovich and Barrows 1984; Gruppen and Frohna 2002).

Constructing a problem representation involves transformation of a patient's specific symptoms and signs into a conceptualization—or representation—of the problem using semantic qualifiers. At this stage, the words reflect meaning the clinician assigns to the case features in relationship to temporal and potential causal relationships between them (Auclair 2007). In other words, students move beyond knowing the words used to describe specific case features to assigning meaning to the words in relationship to case findings—from remembering to understanding—from learning vocabulary to using the vocabulary to represent the clinical problem.

In clinical reasoning, the step of constructing a problem representation occurs between data acquisition and hypothesis generation (Chang et al. 1998). Abstract semantic qualifiers are used to "build a global sense or representation of the problem before tackling possible diagnostic solutions" (Nendaz and Bordage 2002). The problem representation then triggers activation of medical knowledge from long-term memory in the form of plausible diagnoses for the specific case under consideration. Clinicians then purposefully direct further data gathering in relationship to comparing and contrasting diagnostic hypotheses under consideration. Diagnostic accuracy is associated with more thorough and relevant problem representations (Chang et al. 1998).

Generating a problem representation is often an unconscious process (Bowen 2006). Teachers can make this step in the reasoning process explicit by asking students, "what problem are we trying to solve?" Although students at an early stage of learning do not have enough clinical experience to actually solve the clinical problem, students can develop the habit of using clinical vocabulary to construct general problem representations. Feedback on students' problem representations should promote appropriate abstraction of case features using semantic qualifiers and identifying the key attributes—onset, site, severity, chronology, and context—when describing the nature of the clinical problem based on the chief complaint and history of present illness.

Returning to the examples above, the problem representation in Alicia's case could be:

a middle-aged female with a chronic, gradually progressive symmetrical oligoarticular process involving small joints characterized by moderate to severe morning stiffness.

Robert's problem representation might be:

young male with sudden onset of brief, self-limited syncope in the setting of chronic, progressive dyspnea and episodic chest tightness that resolves with rest.

Note in the second example the introduction of additional medical terminology, syncope and dyspnea, that experienced clinicians would use to assign meaning to Robert's problem.

For early clinical learners, we recommend practice with straightforward or typical clinical presentations. Yet, clinical problems are often complex, ill-defined, and ambiguous. In such instances, more than one problem representation simultaneously is possible. Teachers should encourage students to generate appropriate problem representations that may emphasize different key attributes of the case and therefore trigger a broader, yet still plausible set of diagnostic hypotheses for consideration.

Students at this stage of learning often want to know if their problem representations are right or wrong. It is important to point out that construction of a problem representation is an early clinical reasoning step that helps the clinician consider a plausible set of diagnostic hypotheses relevant to the clinical presentation. Each clinician will have her own approach to this conceptualization process influenced by clinical experience. Students should learn that problem representations are not "right or wrong," just "better" when all relevant attributes are addressed using the appropriate semantic qualifiers for the specific clinical problem. Finally, students are often encouraged to summarize their patient's problem at the end of a case presentation. These one-sentence summaries are often called summary statements or assessment statements for a particular patient. These statements are not the same as the problem representation and serve very different purposes in the clinical reasoning process. The problem representation is a more generic formulation of the type of clinical problem to be solved and occurs *early* in the data-gathering process. As further data are purposefully gathered to sort through the diagnostic hypotheses triggered by the problem representation, a more complete and specific picture of the patient's problem is created along with a narrowed plausible differential diagnosis. The summary or assessment statement formulation serves to synthesize these specific characteristics for this patient's problem and sets up a discourse about clinical management or diagnostic testing. Table 4.3 illustrates this process for Robert's clinical presentation. Note how hypothesis-driven inquiry reveals additional clinical information (shown in italics).

Illness Script Mental Repository

Once students have a certain fluency with clinical vocabulary and have learned to conceptualize patients' problems using semantic qualifiers, teachers can introduce an additional structure to help students consider features of a typical diagnosis that includes additional knowledge experienced physicians store in long-term memory. Students will learn to integrate foundational science concepts and pathophysiology with the findings from the clinical history, physical examination, and diagnostic testing.

One format used to describe physicians' mental representations of coherent, causal clinical knowledge used in clinical reasoning is the *illness script* (Custers 2015), first described by Feltovich and Barrows (1984). Illness scripts develop with clinical experience. Custers summarizes the common components of illness scripts as:

> (1) high-level, precompiled, conceptual knowledge structures, which are (2) stored in long-term memory, which (3) represent general (stereotyped) event sequences, in which (4) the individual events are interconnected by temporal and often also causal or hierarchical relationships, that (5) can be activated as integral wholes in appropriate contexts, that (6) contain variables and slots that can be filled with information present in the actual situation, retrieved from memory, or inferred from the context, and that (7) develop as a consequence of routinely performed activities or viewing such activities being performed; in other words, through direct or vicarious experience. (Custers 2015)

Most students in the early years of medical school will not have enough direct or vicarious experience to have begun forming their own full-fledged illness scripts in memory. Nevertheless, as they learn about typical presentations of clinical cases, rudimentary illness scripts begin to form. Junior students with personal experience with an illness may possess a script for it (e.g., "flu" or "motion sickness"). When provided a schema structure that explicitly elicits components of illness scripts, students can organize information about those clinical cases into the structure of illness scripts, taking the vocabulary they are learning and "placing" it in a schema about a particular "typical or exemplar" clinical diagnosis.

4 Prerequisites for Learning Clinical Reasoning

Table 4.3 Evolution of early problem representation to summary statement in the diagnostic reasoning process

Patient's history	Problem representation	Triggered diagnostic hypotheses	Hypothesis-driven inquiry
Robert is a 28-year-old male brought by his friends to the emergency room after he collapsed during the initial part of his first soccer match	Young active male with sudden collapse	Cardiac etiology	Did he lose consciousness?
		Neurologic etiology	
		Intravascular volume loss from trauma	
		Pulmonary embolism	
His friends report loss of consciousness of about 30 s	Young active male with sudden collapse and loss of consciousness	Syncope: cardiac versus neurologic etiology	Was there any involuntary motor activity? Any postictal symptoms?
		Seizure	
No one observed any jerking movements; when he regained consciousness, he was fully alert and aware	Young active male with syncope	Syncope of cardiovascular or neuro-cardiogenic origin	Did he experience any other cardiovascular or neurologic symptoms?
		Vasovagal syncope	
Robert reports difficulty breathing, especially when lying down	Young active male with syncope, dyspnea, and orthopnea	Aortic stenosis	What is the chronology of his respiratory distress?
		Hypertrophic obstructive cardiomyopathy	
		Idiopathic pulmonary arterial hypertension	
		Pulmonary embolism	
He has experienced mild shortness of breath when exercising ever since he can remember, but his symptoms now are a lot worse. *He has not had any palpitations*	Young active male with syncope in the setting of orthopnea and chronic progressive dyspnea	Aortic stenosis	Are there any other cardiovascular symptoms with a similar chronology?
		Hypertrophic obstructive cardiomyopathy	
		Idiopathic pulmonary arterial hypertension	
		Pulmonary embolism	
In retrospect, his exercise tolerance has been declining for the past 9–12 months. He used to be able to do almost anything he wanted but now notices that he gets quite breathless after only a flight of stairs	Young active male with syncope in the setting of orthopnea, chronic progressive severe dyspnea, and declining exercise tolerance	Aortic stenosis	Does he have chest pain?
		Hypertrophic obstructive cardiomyopathy	
		Idiopathic pulmonary arterial hypertension	
		Recurrent pulmonary emboli	

(continued)

Table 4.3 (continued)

Patient's history	Problem representation	Triggered diagnostic hypotheses	Hypothesis-driven inquiry
On two occasions about 4 months ago he had to stop walking upstairs because of chest pain, which scared him. He describes the chest pain as tightness in middle of his chest that never lasts longer than a minute and goes away with rest	Young active male with syncope in the setting of orthopnea, chronic progressive severe dyspnea, declining exercise tolerance, and typical exertional chest pain	Aortic stenosis Hypertrophic obstructive cardiomyopathy Idiopathic pulmonary arterial hypertension Recurrent pulmonary emboli	Does he have any risk factors for pulmonary embolus?
He has not traveled recently (no prolonged immobility), has no history of blood clots, and has no history of malignancy	Young active male with syncope in the setting of orthopnea, chronic progressive severe dyspnea, declining exercise tolerance, and typical exertional chest pain without risk factors for pulmonary embolism	Aortic stenosis Hypertrophic obstructive cardiomyopathy Idiopathic pulmonary arterial hypertension	Does he have preexisting diagnoses (comorbidities) that would make any of the diagnoses under consideration more or less likely?
He remembers he had a heart murmur when he was a child and that when his parents were alive he used to get very painful monthly injections. When he was 18 years old, he took a daily "penicillin" pill, but he has not taken anything for years	Young active male with sudden-onset syncope, chronic progressive dyspnea with orthopnea, intermittent typical chest pain, progressive fatigue, and an unclear history of a heart murmur as a child	Aortic stenosis, probable congenital bicuspid valvular disease Hypertrophic obstructive cardiomyopathy Idiopathic pulmonary arterial hypertension	Hypothesis-driven physical examination is performed
Hypothesis-Driven Physical Examination: Temp of 37.3 °C, HR 125, RR 30, BP 100/50, and oxygen saturation of 89% on room air; JVP is elevated to the angle of the jaw when sitting 45° from supine; carotid pulses diminished with delayed upstroke bilaterally; chest palpation with parasternal heave and precordial thrill; auscultation reveals a 4/6 systolic ejection murmur heard best at the right second intercostal space that does not change with Valsalva maneuver, loud S2, and S3 heard at the apex; peripheral pulses are 1+ and symmetrical; lung auscultation reveals bilateral crackles to level of scapulae; the liver is palpable 3 finger breaths below the right costal margin; skin is cool without cyanosis; 2 + ankle edema noted bilaterally; neurological exam is normal			

(continued)

Table 4.3 (continued)

Patient's history	Problem representation	Triggered diagnostic hypotheses	Hypothesis-driven inquiry
Summary Statement: A 28-year-old male with sudden-onset syncope, moderate to severe dyspnea with orthopnea, in the setting of intermittent chest pain typical of angina, progressive fatigue, and an unclear history of a heart murmur as a child. Exam suggests heart failure. Murmur noted on cardiac auscultation and carotid pulses (*pulsus parvus et tardus*) most suspicious for aortic stenosis. He is at risk for subacute bacterial endocarditis. With a low-grade fever, this should be pursued. A diagnostic echocardiogram will likely be the best approach for distinguishing aortic stenosis from hypertrophic obstructive cardiomyopathy and idiopathic pulmonary arterial hypertension, which are less likely. The echocardiogram would also detect the suspected congenital bicuspid aortic valve abnormality			

Table 4.4 Illness script worksheet

	Attributes	Typical findings
Enabling conditions	Age, sex, race, ethnicity	
	Family history, genetics	
	Habits, exposures, medications	
	Nested comorbidities if any	
Pathophysiological fault		
Clinical consequences	**Onset**	
	Site	
	Severity	
	Chronology	
	Physical exam findings	
	Laboratory findings	
	Imaging findings	

Table 4.4 shows the expanded version of Tables 4.1 and 4.2 as a worksheet for students that provides structure for building knowledge storage in a general mental framework typical of illness scripts. It includes the categorized components of the illness script—enabling (predisposing) conditions, (pathophysiological) fault, and (clinical) consequences—with space for students to record typical features concisely. For *enabling conditions*, students should consider age, sex, race, ethnicity, genetics, nested comorbidities (existing diagnoses with their own illness scripts associated at a lower hierarchical level with the current illness script), environmental exposures, habits (e.g., smoking), and medications; for *pathophysiological fault*, the goal is to integrate science learning with clinical case information to address mechanisms of insult or injury, such as hemodynamic regulation, neuro-regulation, inflammatory process, infectious process, genetic mutation, and metabolic disorder, among others; for *clinical consequences*, the schema builds from the vocabulary training, addressing the chief complaint and history of present illness (onset, site, symptom severity, course/chronology) and adding physical examination findings, laboratory findings, imaging findings, and findings from diagnostic procedures. Of course, not all diagnoses will have information in all of these schema "fields,"

creating opportunities for teachers to emphasize the diagnostic utility of testing and procedures.

Students must gradually build in their long-term memory a mental repository of illness scripts that become readily available for comparison at any new encounter with a patient. This requires elaboration of many cases, with and without guidance. This mental repository can only be built in a curriculum that provides many own or vicarious encounters with patients, real or simulated, and that stimulates students to study and reflect on these cases.

Contrastive Learning

Contrastive learning "involves prompting the learner to explicitly search for similarities and differences between problems" (Ark et al. 2007). Applying the concept of analogical transfer whereby learners address novel problems with strategies used to solve similar problems previously, Ark and colleagues demonstrated superior diagnostic accuracy for contrastive learning compared to traditional serial learning. They trained novices to identify key features of a series of typical abnormal electrocardiograms (ECG), to compare and contrast abnormal features of the initial ECG with a normal ECG and with an ECG typical of a plausible alternative diagnosis. The goal was to assist students with learning the critical features that discriminate between categories by having them intentionally consider similarities and differences between pairs of abnormal ECG exemplars. When compared to novices instructed to learn key features of exemplar ECGs in a serial, non-contrastive way, students instructed in a contrastive learning strategy identified the correct ECG diagnosis significantly more often. Others have recommended using a compare and contrast approach to learning with a focus on deep learning of a limited number of prototypical clinical presentations related to a single problem representation in order to create strong anchors in memory (Bordage 1994).

Thus, the next step in preparing early medical students for clinical reasoning involves contrastive learning. Once students have learned to develop schemas for the clinical cases under discussion, teachers can introduce the concept of the differential diagnosis and the process of comparing and contrasting a limited number of diagnostic considerations. For any given problem representation formulated from information revealed early in the clinical case, at least two plausible diagnostic hypotheses are selected for comparison. Preselection, as opposed to student selection, of the diagnoses to be considered is important at this stage of learning. Diagnostic possibilities must be realistic and easily distinguishable. Thus, for Alicia's case, one would choose to have the students compare the exemplar case of rheumatoid arthritis with that of osteoarthritis as shown in Table 4.5. Once the schemas for individual clinical presentations are described, putting the two side by side as shown allows students to compare and contrast the differences and learn to identify the distinguishing features.

Table 4.5 Contrasting competing illness scripts

		Example of a problem representation	
		A middle-aged female with a chronic, gradually progressive symmetrical oligoarticular process involving small joints characterized by moderate to severe morning stiffness	
Exemplar diagnosis		1- Osteoarthritis	2- Rheumatoid arthritis
Enabling conditions	Age, sex, race, ethnicity	Over 50 yrs.; either sex	30–60 years, F:M ratio 3:1
	Family history, genetics	+/− family history	+ family history; shared epitope, HLA-DRB1
	Habits, exposures, medications	None	Smoking
	Nested comorbidities	None	Coronary artery disease
Pathophysiological fault		Mechanical, degenerative; cartilage breakdown and subsequent bone hypertrophy	Inflammatory, immunologic; synovitis, pannus and subsequent erosion of juxta-articular bone
Clinical consequences	**Onset**	Gradual	Gradual
	Site	Small, large joints; appendicular; polyarticular; involves DIP	Small, large joints; appendicular; polyarticular; usually spares DIP
	Severity	Mild	Moderate
	Chronology	Chronic persistent	Chronic persistent
	Exam findings	Boney enlargement of joint; mild tenderness if any	Warmth; erythema; tenderness; swelling; occasional rheumatoid nodules
	Laboratory findings	None	Elevated ESR; rheumatoid factor anti-CCP
	Imaging findings	Sclerosis of bone under cartilage; joint space narrowing; osteophytes	Erosive polyarthritis; joint space narrowing

Hypothesis-Driven Inquiry

In traditional medical education, preclinical medical students learn components of the physical examination and then learn to assemble these components into a logical sequence necessary for the head-to-toe examination of any patient (Nendaz and Bordage 2002; Yudkowsky et al. 2009). Except perhaps for the purpose of documenting a baseline examination in a healthy person, this approach to learning the physical examination does not promote its purpose as a data-gathering step in the clinical reasoning process. Such decontextualized learning delays comprehension of the significance of abnormal examination findings as discriminating features in the diagnostic process. As Yudkowsky and colleagues suggest, "students do not learn to appreciate how an abnormal finding would appear or what it might mean." These authors studied an alternative approach designed to support contextual learning by embedding instruction in physical examination maneuvers within diagnostic reasoning tasks. The approach emphasizes students' abilities to anticipate which examination maneuvers will help discriminate between diagnostic considerations and to recognize diagnostically useful examination findings. A useful guide is available for implementing this method (Nishigori et al. 2011).

Similarly, Hasnain and colleagues studied the relationship between history-taking behaviors, semantic versus symptom-driven discourse, and diagnostic accuracy. Four interviewing behaviors were associated with high diagnostic accuracy: thorough exploration of the patient's chief complaint early in the clinical encounter, asking questions in close proximity (illustrative of a line of reasoning about a diagnostic hypothesis), asking patients to provide further clarifying information, and summarizing information gathered during the interview. The authors describe these behaviors as "purposeful or hypothesis-driven inquiry" (Hasnain et al. 2001). Table 4.3 illustrates this process for Robert's clinical problem.

Diagnostic Verification

Diagnostic verification is defined by Kassirer et al. as "the process in which one or more hypotheses are accepted as sufficiently valid to permit further decision making" (Kassirer et al. 2010) and is referred to by Gruppen and Frohna as evaluation ("guiding the acquisition of additional information and, eventually, the decision to stop the cycle and move on to action") (Gruppen and Frohna 2002). We suggest including in the definition of diagnostic verification *all actions that lead to confirmation of the correctness, to the extent possible, of the final diagnosis* even if only to learn from a case and to store a case in memory, contributing to an enriched personal repository of illness scripts. As the skill of clinical reasoning is highly dependent on this repository, any solidification should enhance this skill. In clinical training, given duty hour restrictions, short patient stays, and frequent patient handovers, diagnostic verification—finding out about the consequences of one's diagnostic reasoning process—does not always happen and may need active effort on top of regular clinical duties. Preclinical students should start developing the habit of diagnostic verification, as that will enhance the retrieval of patient cases and enriched illness scripts from long-term memory in the future.

How Does the CBCR Method Address These Prerequisites?

While this chapter is not focused on the description of the CBCR method, it is useful to consider to what extent the CBCR method, described more extensively in Part II, reinforces the prerequisite skills for clinical reasoning. Table 4.6 shows how that is the case.

In summary, introducing concepts associated with strong clinical reasoning performance early in medical school, described here as prerequisites for clinical reasoning, provides an alternative approach to preparing students for their immersive clinical experiences. Learning the clinical vocabulary physicians use when presenting and discussing clinical cases prepares students to become members of the knowledge community of clinical medicine. Learning to translate patients' chief complaint and history of present illness into abstract summaries using semantic qualifiers prepares students to describe thorough and accurate problem representations, an important step in diagnostic reasoning. Abstracting and recording key clinical information into a schema aligning with illness script formation helps students to associate key clinical attributes with pathophysiological explanations of disease processes in the context of clinical cases and store these as units in long-

Table 4.6 Relating the prerequisites to the CBCR method

Prerequisite element	Relationship to CBCR
Clinical vocabulary	As a method that requires active oral participation in reasoning by all students, CBCR provides excellent opportunities to practice the use of medical vocabulary
Problem representation	Many CBCR cases introduce the encounter in the patient's words and have as a first assignment for students "what is, in your own words, the reason for the encounter?" or "what is the chief complaint?" Questions like this force students to represent the problem in a structured way, preparing students for creating problem representations using abstract semantic qualifiers
Illness script mental repository	The background of the CBCR method actually is to engage junior medical students in the creation of mental constructs of a limited number of prototypical diagnoses to serve as a framework for early comparing and contrasting of patterns
Contrastive learning	One dominant approach during all CBCR cases is the creation and completion of two-dimensional tables on a blackboard or flipchart, with findings on one axis and diagnostic hypotheses on the other. With plusses and minuses, student groups must continuously contrast the likelihood of diagnoses using findings from the history, physical examination, and tests
Hypothesis-driven inquiry	A feature of the CBCR method is that gradually more information about cases is revealed and students are asked to respond to new information by suggesting new hypothesis or new information needed. By nature, CBCR cases stimulate hypothesis-driven inquiry
Diagnostic verification	As all cases eventually end with one diagnosis, CBCR cases naturally include diagnostic verification. The drawback is that students do not need to be stimulated to pursue that information. Training of that habit is more logical in the clinical environment than in the classroom setting

term memory. Comparing side-by-side schemas for plausible diagnostic considerations related to a specific case and problem representation reinforces for students the important step of contrastive thinking. Learning to consider the history and physical examination as important steps in data acquisition that help physicians to discriminate between diagnostic possibilities and pursuing diagnostic verification bring all of these prerequisites together to prepare students for application of these skills as they develop competence in clinical reasoning.

References

Aper, L., Reniers, J., Derese, A., & Veldhuijzen, W. (2014). Managing the complexity of doing it all: An exploratory study on students' experiences when trained stepwise in conducting consultations. *BMC Medical Education, 14*(1), 206. http://doi.org/10.1186/1472-6920-14-206

Ark, T. K., Brooks, L. R., & Eva, K. W. (2007). The benefits of flexibility: The pedagogical value of instructions to adopt multifaceted diagnostic reasoning strategies. *Medical Education, 41*(3), 281–287. http://doi.org/10.1111/j.1365-2929.2007.02688.x

Auclair, F. (2007). Problem formulation by medical students: An observation study. *BMC Medical Education, 7*(1), 16. http://doi.org/10.1186/1472-6920-7-16

Barrows, H., & Tamblyn, R. (1980). *Problem-based learning*. New York: Springer Publishing Company.

Bordage, G., & Lemieux, M. (1991). Semantic structures and diagnostic thinking of experts and novices. *Academic Medicine, 66*(9), S70–S72. http://doi.org/10.1097/00001888-199109000-00045

Bordage, G., Connell, K., Chang, R., Gecht, M., & Sinacore, J. (1997). Assessing the semantic content of clinical case presentations: Studies of reliability and concurrent validity. *Academic Medicine, 72*(10), S37–S39.

Bordage, G. (1994). Elaborated knowledge: A key to successful diagnostic thinking. *Academic Medicine, 69*(11), 883–885.

Bowen, J. L. (2006). Educational strategies to promote clinical diagnostic reasoning. *The New England Journal of Medicine, 355*(21), 2217–2225.

Chang, R., Bordage, G., & Connell, K. (1998). The importance of early problem representation during case presentations. *Academic Emergency Medicine: Official Journal of the Society for Academic Emergency Medicine, 73*(10), S109–S111.

Cook, D. A., Erwin, P. J., & Triola, M. M. (2010). Computerized virtual patients in health professions education: A systematic review and meta-analysis. *Academic Medicine, 85*(10), 1589–1602.

Cooke, M., Irby, D., & O'Brien, B. C. (2010). *Educating physicians – A call for reform of medical school and residency*. Hoboken: Jossey-Bass/Carnegie Foundation for the Advancement of Teaching.

Custers, E. J. F. M. (2015). Thirty years of illness scripts: Theoretical origins and practical applications. *Medical Teacher, 37*(5), 457–462.

Feltovich, P., & Barrows, H. (1984). Issues of generality in medical problem solving. In H. G. Schmidt & M. L. de Voider (Eds.), *Tutorials in problem-based learning: A new direction in teaching the health professions* (pp. 128–142). Assen: Van Gorcum.

Gruppen, L., & Frohna, A. (2002). Clinical reasoning. In G. Norman, C. Van der Vleuten, & D. Newble (Eds.), *International handbook of research in medical education* (pp. 205–230). Dordrecht: Kluwer Academic Publishers.

Hasnain, M., Bordage, G., Connell, K. J., & Sinacore, J. M. (2001). History-taking behaviors associated with diagnostic competence of clerks: An exploratory study. *Academic Medicine, 76*(10 Suppl), S14–S17.

Jacobson, K., Fisher, D. L., Hoffman, K., & Tsoulas, K. D. (2010). Integrated cases section: A course designed to promote clinical reasoning in year 2 medical students. *Teaching and Learning in Medicine, 22*(4), 312–316.

Kassirer, J., Wong, J., & Kopelman, R. (2010). *Learning clinical reasoning* (2nd ed.). Baltimore: Lippincott Williams & Wilkins.

Kim, K.-J., & Kee, C. (2012). Evaluation of an e-PBL model to promote individual reasoning. *Medical Teacher, 35*(3), e978–e983.

LaRochelle, J., Gilliland, W., Torre, D., Baker, E. A., Mechaber, A. J., Poremba, J., & Durning, S. (2009). Readdressing the need for consensus in preclinical education. *Military Medicine, 174*(10), 1081–1087.

Nendaz, M. R., & Bordage, G. (2002). Promoting diagnostic problem representation. *Medical Education, 36*(8), 760–766.

Nishigori, H., Masuda, K., Kikukawa, M., Kawashima, A., Yudkowsky, R., Bordage, G., & Otaki, J. (2011). A model teaching session for the hypothesis-driven physical examination. *Medical Teacher, 33*(5), 410–417.

O'Brien, B. C., & Poncelet, A. N. (2010). Transition to clerkship courses : Preparing students to enter the workplace. *Academic Medicine, 85*(12), 1862–1869. http://doi.org/10.1097/ACM.0b013e3181fa2353

Skeff, K. M. (2014). Reassessing the HPI: The chronology of present illness (CPI). *Journal of General Internal Medicine, 29*(1), 13–15.

Yudkowsky, R., Otaki, J., Lowenstein, T., Riddle, J., Nishigori, H., & Bordage, G. (2009). A hypothesis-driven physical examination learning and assessment procedure for medical students: Initial validity evidence. *Medical Education, 43*(8), 729–740.

Open Access This chapter is licensed under the terms of the Creative Commons Attribution 4.0 International License (http://creativecommons.org/licenses/by/4.0/), which permits use, sharing, adaptation, distribution and reproduction in any medium or format, as long as you give appropriate credit to the original author(s) and the source, provide a link to the Creative Commons license and indicate if changes were made.

The images or other third party material in this chapter are included in the chapter's Creative Commons license, unless indicated otherwise in a credit line to the material. If material is not included in the chapter's Creative Commons license and your intended use is not permitted by statutory regulation or exceeds the permitted use, you will need to obtain permission directly from the copyright holder.

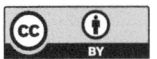

Chapter 5
Approaches to Assessing the Clinical Reasoning of Preclinical Students

Olle ten Cate and Steven J. Durning

If clinical reasoning is considered critical for any physician and an ability a student should acquire during undergraduate medical education, then educators should attempt to assess whether students satisfactorily meet this objective.

In earlier chapters we have establish that clinical reasoning has two components: analytic reasoning and nonanalytic reasoning (i.e., pattern recognition). Hence these two may be the focus of assessment: (1) Do students understand physiology and the pathophysiologic mechanisms and enabling conditions that lead to disease and consequently recognize signs and symptoms observable in patients? and (2) Do students build a mental repository of illness scripts that allow them to recognize patterns in the patients they encounter?

Clearly these objectives require substantial medical knowledge and substantial experience in patient care. And if clinical reasoning by definition, as some say, must include the context in which the physicians works (Woods and Mylopoulos 2015), how reasonable is it to test preclinical student on their clinical reasoning ability? According to Bowen and Ilgen, diagnostic reasoning is not a discrete, enduring, or reliably measurable skill. Accurate measurement in fact requires an observer to interpret processes that are heavily context dependent, usually not explicitly articulated, and often occur below conscious awareness of the observed clinician (Bowen and Ilgen 2014). Nevertheless, authors have attempted to infer progress in clinical reasoning ability across years using a written progress test (Williams et al. 2011).

O. ten Cate (✉)
Center for Research and Development of Education, University Medical Center Utrecht, Utrecht, The Netherlands
e-mail: T.J.tenCate@umcutrecht.nl

S.J. Durning
Uniformed Services University of the Health Sciences, Bethesda, MD, USA
e-mail: steven.durning@usuhs.edu

© The Author(s) 2018
O. ten Cate et al. (eds.), *Principles and Practice of Case-based Clinical Reasoning Education*, Innovation and Change in Professional Education 15, https://doi.org/10.1007/978-3-319-64828-6_5

Case-based clinical reasoning education, or any other approach recommended for preclinical education, attempts to prepare students for clinical encounters. While assessing clinical reasoning *in context* may not be reasonable for these students, a more limited approach, using written test approaches, is possible. Analytic reasoning is practiced in basic science or integrated courses, and pattern recognition ability may already be acquired on a very basic level. The CBCR course, as described in Part II of this book, has the deliberate intention to help students build a limited illness script mental repository for a number of common medical conditions including the differential diagnosis of adjacent conditions. This can be the focus of a test.

Without mentioning the word validity, these introductory sentences pertain to validity. The validity of educational and psychological tests has been reconceptualized in the past decades by scholars such as Messick and Kane (Cook et al. 2015). The validity of a test should be argued from the perspective of the content, response process, internal structure, relationship to other variables, and consequences of the test (AERA/APA/NCME 2014; Downing 2003). For clinical reasoning in preclinical students, the consequences should be the readiness to encounter patients in the clinical setting. The content should focus on important knowledge to allow analytic reasoning as can be expected in such encounters and for the recognition of patterns they have encountered in preclinical education. Response processes, or the way questions in such tests are asked, should resemble the clinical thinking pathways that happen in such encounters and the relationship to other variables may be a hindsight evaluation whether students with a high score indeed seem to do well in clinical reasoning in practice. While we have stressed the limitations in clinical reasoning that must be faced in the preclinical period, it is important to simulate situations they will face once they assume patient-related clinical tasks. As assessment is a powerful stimulus for learning, tests should be designed in such a way that students spend their energy optimally in anticipation of clinical encounters.

Current Methods of Assessing Clinical Reasoning

Educators looking for methods to assess clinical reasoning will find most recommended approaches to be used in clinical education, such as at the bedside, and only few focusing on the testing of reasoning in the preclinical phase, e.g., in a written test format. In terms of Miller's four-level pyramid of assessment in medical education (knows – knows how – shows how – does), the highest three are all to some extent suitable for the assessment of clinical reasoning (Miller 1990). A "knows how" test would present a patient case and asks the candidate to arrive at a diagnosis and/or a therapy. During a "shows how" test, an examiner would ask the student to clinically reason in a standardized patient encounter such as during an objective structured clinical examination (OSCE), and an assessment at the "does" level would ask a student to reason related to a real patient case in the hospital. Table 5.1 summarizes some frequently used, or specifically designed, methods to assess clinical

Table 5.1 Approaches to the assessment of clinical reasoning from the literature

Miller level	Format	Specific methods	Selected references
Knows	[While knowledge is essential for clinical reasoning, factual knowledge tests per se are less suitable to assess clinical reasoning]		
Knows how	Written or electronic format	Constructed response methods	
		Short-answer open questions' test	Rademakers et al. (2005)
		Clinical reasoning problems' test	Groves et al. (2002)
		Written case summaries	Dory et al. (2016)
		Forced choice methods	
		Extended matching questions' test	Case and Swanson (1998)
		Script concordance test	Charlin et al. (2000)
		Comprehensive integrative puzzle test	Ber (2003)
		Case-based clinical reasoning test	See Chap. 7
Shows how	Standardized simulation format	Standardized patient station in an objective structured clinical examination (OSCE)	Sloane et al. (1995) and Hawkins and Boulet (2008)
		Patient assessment and management examination (PAME)	Macrae et al. (2000)
Does	Oral format	Chart-stimulated recall and case-based discussion (CSR/CBD)	Tekian and Yudkowsky (2007) and Singh and Norcini (2013)
		Standardized oral examination	Tekian and Yudkowsky (2007) and Norcini and Burch (2007)
		Mini clinical evaluation exercise	

reasoning with reference to Miller's Pyramid. In addition to this list, a specific test format has been developed for CBCR courses, which is discussed in Chap. 7.

For preclinical students, Miller's levels of *shows how* and *does* are less applicable. To assess students' clinical reasoning ability in students before they encounter patients, a written or electronic test format is more suitable for several reasons. Cohort of students can be tested at once, standards can be set, and reliable scores can be generated. One can argue that clinical reasoning should ideally measure actual performance. That would yield the best construct alignment between the goals and objectives, what is taught, and what is tested.

For CBCR courses with large numbers of students a written, or preferably an electronic, test format is recommended to establish a reliable examination. In a recent literature review on question types for clinical reasoning tests suitable for electronic tests, Van Bruggen and colleagues identified eight types (van Bruggen et al. 2012): script concordance test questions, extended matching questions, comprehensive integrative puzzle questions, modified essay/short-answer questions, long-menu questions, multiple-choice questions, and true/false questions. The latter two were identified as least suitable, and we added two formats, all briefly discussed in Table 5.2. Features from different formats have been combined in the CBCR test format explained more extensively in Chap. 7.

Table 5.2 Questions suitable for written or electronic assessment of clinical reasoning ability

Question type	Item and tests' description	Features and comment
Script concordance test items (Charlin et al. 2000; Lubarsky et al. 2011)	A short patient vignette is given + a diagnostic hypothesis. Next, a new finding is presented. The candidate must score how this finding renders the hypothesis (much) less to (much) more likely, on a scale from −2 to +2, with score 0 being "no change"	Model answers are constructed using a panel of experts answering the questions. As they may disagree, a weighting is applied to scale values based on the number of experts choosing that value
		SCT is widely used but is also criticized for its validity and practicality (van den Broek et al. 2012; Lineberry et al. 2013)
Modified essay or short-answer questions (Rademakers et al. 2005)	Short-answer case-based questions that result in reliable tests have a short case vignette, require an answer of no more than 20 words (preferably much less), have predetermined model answers and scoring instructions to guide correction, and yield a scaled score (e.g., 0–3 points)	Experience learns that 40–50 questions should make a reliable test (ten Cate 1997)
		The major drawback of SAQs is that they require hand scoring, which may take time, specifically if there are many students
Clinical reasoning problems (Groves et al. 2002)	CRP questions contain a case vignette and ask for (a) a most likely diagnosis and (b) features from the vignette that support or oppose the hypothesis, each with a weighting (1–3), (c) an alternative diagnosis with (d) similar follow-up question as b	Groves et al. report satisfactory reliability and construct and external validity with a voluntary 10 CRP test, but without test conditions (Groves et al. 2002)
		The major drawback of CRPs is that they require hand scoring, which may take time, specifically if there are many students
Extended matching questions (Case and Swanson 1998)	EMQs have a theme (e.g., "fatigue"), a list of options (e.g., 10–20 diagnoses or lab results), a lead question ("what is the most likely diagnosis?" "which lab result do you expect?"), and then two or more case vignettes	Used by the National Board of Medical Examiners, EMQs are well known in the United States; less so outside the United States
		Number of EMQs and testing time required for a reliable test (up to 100 items and 4 hours) is quite large (Beullens et al. 2002)

(continued)

Table 5.2 (continued)

Question type	Item and tests' description	Features and comment
Comprehensive integrative puzzle test CIP (Ber 2003)	One CIP is a table of 4*4–6*6 cells with in the first column a series of related (differential) diagnoses. Other columns are headed *history, physical examination, test results, X-ray, management*, or similar. Empty cells must be filled from separate option lists to construct, horizontally, logical illness scripts. The sum of correct cells yields a score	Four to five CIP cells may constitute a reliable test. Construct validity has been established (Groothoff et al. 2008)
		A potential drawback is the difficulty of item writing. A too narrow differential diagnosis column may make the construction of valid option lists hard; a too diverse differential diagnosis column may make CIP too easy
Long-menu questions (Schuwirth et al. 1996)	Long-menu questions are used in electronic testing as an alternative for open questions and have a very long list of options to eliminate guessing. Advanced formats match typed-in questions with the list to enable automatic scoring	A drawback is that more than one entry word is difficult to recognize automatically, and mistakes can be made if multiple words are required. In addition, the same drawbacks as with multiple-choice questions apply, without the cueing disadvantage
Written case summaries (Dory et al. 2016)	Candidates receive multiple case vignettes describing in lay language a patient's history of present illness, past medical history, and physical examination findings. They must summarize the case as they would present to an attending staff, in a few sentences using medical terminology (semantic qualifiers) to measure problem representation. Answers are scored using a 3-item rubric focusing on pertinent findings, semantic quality, and a global rating	This approach aligns well with Bowen's prerequisites for clinical reasoning (Chap. 4). The authors report "good evidence regarding scoring and generalizability" in a study with 8 case summary questions among 700 medical students, but acceptable reliability may require more cases. The method may be part of a battery of different items. Scoring time per rater is estimated 1 min per case, and rater training may be needed. Technology may assist the rating in the future

Almost all of the test forms in Table 5.2 use a key-feature approach. Key-feature questions focus on critical steps in the solution of a clinical problem and may pertain to aspects that learners generally find difficult or that are critical in patient management (Page et al. 1995). The development of the key-feature approach in the 1990s was a move away from the traditional assessment of clinical reasoning using a comprehensive examination of a patient management problem (Page and Bordage 1995). A recent review reconfirmed the generally favorable psychometric properties of question types derived from the key-feature approach (Hrynchak et al. 2014).

In this chapter, we have provided a brief overview of current methods assessment of clinical reasoning, with a focus on methods suitable for preclinical students in a written fashion. We acknowledge this overview is limited. An excellent recent overview of more clinically oriented approaches was provided by Rencic and colleagues (2016). In addition, many studies have been conducted to measure clinical reasoning ability, and several of these have used experimental outcome measures that might be suitable for standard assessment at some time. Computer-based tests (Kunina-Habenicht et al. 2015), virtual reality assessment (Forsberg et al. 2016), eye-tracking (Kok and Jarodzka 2017), neuroimaging (Durning et al. 2015), and other sophisticated methods require however further evaluation before they translate to established and feasible methods, meeting Van der Vleuten's utility criteria of reliability, validity, cost-effectiveness, educational impact and acceptability, and other useful measures of quality (van der Vleuten and Schuwirth 2005).

References

AERA/APA/NCME. (2014). In B. Plake, L. Wise, et al. (Eds.), *Standards for educational and psychological testing*. Washington, DC: American Educational Research Association.
Ber, R. (2003). The CIP (comprehensive integrative puzzle) assessment method. *Medical Teacher, 25*(2), 171–176.
Beullens, J., et al. (2002). Are extended-matching multiple-choice items appropriate for a final test in medical education? *Medical Teacher, 24*(4), 390–395.
Bowen, J. L., & Ilgen, J. S. (2014). Now you see it, now you don't: What thinking aloud tells us about clinical reasoning. *Journal of Graduate Medical Education, 6,* 783–785.
Broek, W. E. S., et al. (2012). Effects of two different instructional formats on scores and reliability of a script concordance test. *Perspectives on Medical Education, 1*(3), 119–128.
Case, S. M., & Swanson, D. B. (1998). *Constructing written test questions for the basic and clinical sciences* (2nd ed.). Philadelphia: National Board of Medical Examiners.
Charlin, B., et al. (2000). The script concordance test: A tool to assess the reflective clinician. *Teaching and Learning in Medicine, 12*(4), 189–195.
Cook, D. A., et al. (2015). A contemporary approach to validity arguments: A practical guide to Kane's framework. *Medical Education, 49*(6), 560–575.
Dory, V., et al. (2016). In brief: Validity of case summaries in written examinations of clinical reasoning. *Teaching and Learning in Medicine, 0*(0), 1–10. Available at: http://ezproxy.usherbrooke.ca/login?url=https://search.ebscohost.com/login.aspx?direct=true&db=mnh&AN=27294400&site=ehost-live
Downing, S. M. (2003). Validity: On the meaningful interpretation of assessment data. *Medical Education, 37*(9), 830–837.
Durning, S. J., et al. (2015). Neural basis of nonanalytical reasoning expertise during clinical evaluation. *Brain and Behaviour, 309,* 1–10.
Forsberg, E., et al. (2016). Assessing progression of clinical reasoning through virtual patients: An exploratory study. *Nurse Education in Practice, 16*(1), 97–103.

Groothoff, J. W., et al. (2008). Growth of analytical thinking skills over time as measured with the MATCH test. *Medical Education, 42*(10), 1037–1043.

Groves, M., Scott, I., & Alexander, H. (2002). Assessing clinical reasoning: A method to monitor its development in a PBL curriculum. *Medical Teacher, 24*(5), 507–515.

Hawkins, R. E., & Boulet, J. R. (2008). Direct observation: Standardized patients. In E. S. Holmboe & R. E. Hawkins (Eds.), *Practical guide to the evaluation of clinical competence* (pp. 102–118). Philadelphia: Mosby Elsevier.

Hrynchak, P., Glover Takahashi, S., & Nayer, M. (2014). Key-feature questions for assessment of clinical reasoning: A literature review. *Medical Education, 48*(9), 870–883.

Kok, E. M., & Jarodzka, H. (2017). Before your very eyes: The value and limitations of eye tracking in medical education. *Medical Education, 51*(1), 114–122.

Kunina-Habenicht, O., et al. (2015). Assessing clinical reasoning (ASCLIRE): Instrument development and validation. *Advances in Health Sciences Education, 20*(5), 1205–1224.

Lineberry, M., Kreiter, C. D., & Bordage, G. (2013). Threats to validity in the use and interpretation of script concordance test scores. *Medical Education, 47*(12), 1175–1183.

Lubarsky, S., et al. (2011). Script concordance testing: A review of published validity evidence. *Medical Education, 45*(4), 329–338.

Macrae, H., et al. (2000). A comprehensive examination for senior surgical residents. *American Journal of Surgery, 179*, 190–193.

Miller, G. E. (1990). The assessment of clinical skills/competence/performance. *Academic Medicine, 87*(7), S63–S67.

Norcini, J., & Burch, V. (2007). Workplace-based assessment as an educational tool: AMEE guide no. 31. *Medical Teacher, 29*(9), 855–871.

Page, G., & Bordage, G. (1995). The Medical Council of Canada's key features project: A more valid written examination of clinical decision-making skills. *Academe, 70*(2), 104–110.

Page, G., Bordage, G., & Allen, T. (1995). Developing key-feature problems and examinations to assess clinical decision-making skills. *Academic Medicine, 70*, 194–201.

Rademakers, J., ten Cate, O., & Bär, P. R. (2005). Progress testing with short answer questions. *Medical Teacher, 27*(7), 578–582.

Rencic, J., et al. (2016). Understanding the assessment of clinical reasoning. In P. Wimmers & M. Mentkowski (Eds.), *Assessing competence in professional performance across disciplines and professions* (pp. 209–235). Cham: Springer International Publishing.

Schuwirth, L. W., et al. (1996). Computerized long-menu questions as an alternative to open-ended questions in computerized assessment. *Medical Education, 30*(1), 50–55.

Singh, T., & Norcini, J. (2013). Workplace-based assessment. In W. McGaghie (Ed.), *International best practices for evaluation in the health professions* (pp. 257–279). London: Radcliffe Publishing Ltd.

Sloane, D., et al. (1995). The objective structured clinical examination. The new gold standard for evaluating. *Annals of Surgery, 222*(6), 735–742.

Tekian, A., & Yudkowsky, R. (2007). Oral examinations. In S. Downing & R. Yudkowsky (Eds.), *Assessment in health professions education* (pp. 269–286). New York: Routledge.

ten Cate, O. (1997). In A. Scherpbier et al. (Eds.), *Comparing reliabilities of true/false and short-answer questions in written problem solving tests* (pp. 193–196). Dordrecht: Kluwer Academic Publishers.

van Bruggen, L., et al. (2012). Preferred question types for computer-based assessment of clinical reasoning: A literature study. *Perspectives on Medical Education, 1*(4), 162–171.

van der Vleuten, C. P. M., & Schuwirth, L. W. T. (2005). Assessing professional competence: From methods to programmes. *Medical Education, 39*(3), 309–317.

Williams, R. G., et al. (2011). Tracking development of clinical reasoning ability across five medical schools using a progress test. *Academic Medicine: Journal of the Association of American Medical Colleges, 86*(9), 1148–1154.

Woods, N. N., & Mylopoulos, M. (2015). On clinical reasoning research and applications: Redefining expertise. *Medical Education, 49*(5), 543–543.

Open Access This chapter is licensed under the terms of the Creative Commons Attribution 4.0 International License (http://creativecommons.org/licenses/by/4.0/), which permits use, sharing, adaptation, distribution and reproduction in any medium or format, as long as you give appropriate credit to the original author(s) and the source, provide a link to the Creative Commons license and indicate if changes were made.

The images or other third party material in this chapter are included in the chapter's Creative Commons license, unless indicated otherwise in a credit line to the material. If material is not included in the chapter's Creative Commons license and your intended use is not permitted by statutory regulation or exceeds the permitted use, you will need to obtain permission directly from the copyright holder.

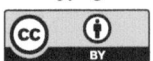

Part II
The Method of Case-Based Clinical Reasoning Education

Chapter 6
Case-Based Clinical Reasoning in Practice

Angela van Zijl, Maria van Loon, and Olle ten Cate

Following the summary description of CBCR education in Chap. 1, this chapter elaborates on a CBCR course in practice. This is to provide teachers and curriculum developers as much as possible with a detailed picture of a CBCR course as it unfolds. The description is derived from many years of experience at UMC Utrecht, which can be at some variance with other sites using CBCR, but readers should read this with their own local constraints in mind and adapt as far as necessary to meet local needs.

The Course Conditions

Scheduling Groups

CBCR takes place in small groups consisting of 10–13 students. If the class consists of 300 students (as is the case in Utrecht), 24 groups operate in parallel with 12 or 13 students each, which is a convenient number of groups to schedule from a logistical point of view. If all groups must meet within a week, 1 or 2 days can be allocated to schedule four sets of six groups for a CBCR session (e.g., groups 1–6

A. van Zijl (✉)
Wilhelmina's Children Hospital, Utrecht, The Netherlands
e-mail: angela_van_zijl@hotmail.com

M. van Loon
University Medical Center Utrecht, Utrecht, The Netherlands
e-mail: mariavloon@gmail.com

O. ten Cate
Center for Research and Development of Education, University Medical Center Utrecht, Utrecht, The Netherlands
e-mail: T.J.tenCate@umcutrecht.nl

© The Author(s) 2018
O. ten Cate et al. (eds.), *Principles and Practice of Case-based Clinical Reasoning Education*, Innovation and Change in Professional Education 15,
https://doi.org/10.1007/978-3-319-64828-6_6

and 7–12 from 9:00-11:00 and 11:00–13:00, respectively, and groups 13–18 and 19–24 in the afternoon or at the same time the next day). This way the same rooms and consultants can be scheduled for multiple groups, and at the same time the exchange of information can be avoided by preventing too much spreading in between groups. Avoidance of exchange of information is to maximize the freshness of the case for the students. During the session follow-up information about the patient is provided that should not be known before the session.

Spread of Sessions Over the Year

Ten CBCR meetings in a year is a convenient number, but it could be twice as many. This can be scheduled, with at least 2 weeks in between sessions, to allow for enough time for students, consultants, and particularly peer teachers (see participant roles) to prepare for sessions.

Curriculum planners should be mindful of conflicting obligations of the students for other courses and avoid planning sessions just before examinations. Another important consideration in planning sessions is that CBCR tries to apply and rehearse previously acquired knowledge. A case of a patient with shortness of breath should, for all groups, be scheduled *after* student had education about physiology and anatomy, and preferably pathology of relevant organ systems, in this case the respiratory system.

Rooms, Arrangement and Facilities

Rooms are suitable for CBCR session if students face each other and their peer teachers. A recommended arrangement is a square placement of tables with 2–4 chairs on each side. Peer teachers best sit next to each other and the consultant at a corner, to stress their more aloof role during the session. There should either be a blackboard (or whiteboard) or a flip-over chart if there is no board. A board is necessary to build clinical reasoning when filling tables of diagnostic hypotheses and history, signs and symptoms, test results, etc. in an interactive dialogue with the group.

Increasingly, computer projection screens are used, for instance, to depict the text of a "handout" about new patient information at requested moments during the session. The table filling during group dialogues can also be done starting with an empty table on a projection screen. But an old-fashioned blackboard is at least as convenient.

Consultants

Consultants, the teachers present, should be clinicians and can be recruited from various clinical departments. They do not necessarily have to be very experienced clinicians. Indeed, that may even be a drawback. An experienced subspecialist may have less fresh knowledge about cases outside their specialty than a recent graduate. Our experiences with educationally interested residents or even interns around graduation, serving preclinical student groups, are excellent (Zijdenbos et al. 2010, 2011). Sometimes CBCR sessions are held with more advanced medical student groups; then a more experienced clinician may be advisable as a consultant.

It can be recommended, for reasons of group dynamics, to have a similar consultant facilitate a group throughout a year. The detailed consultant version of case descriptions includes answers to all questions and will support any physician to guide a CBCR session with junior medical students in cases that are not their specialty.

Materials

The written materials of a CBCR case include three versions: (a) a student version with the objectives, the requirements, a case introduction, and questions; (b) a peer teacher version, including all information of the student version and with additional information, hints, and all hand-out texts about additional patient information that needs to be provided at the right time during the session; and (c) a consultant version, consisting of the peer teacher version supplemented with background information and all model answers.

All students receive all student cases, usually together at the beginning of the course. Downloadable texts are convenient. At each session, the consultant provides the upcoming peer teachers with the peer teacher version of the case of the next session.

A CBCR Session

A CBCR session has a minimum duration of 1'45" h and a maximum of 2'30" h. During a session usually one but sometimes two patient cases are being discussed. The session is preferably led by three peer teachers. Having two peer teachers doing this is not impossible, but one peer teacher is not recommended as that makes sessions too vulnerable, and more than three is not practical. Before a meeting, all students should have read the assigned literature about the topic of the case described in a *student version* of the case that they have received at the beginning of the year or at least sufficiently long before the session. Clinical practice guidelines and a handbook for general practice could be suitable as preparatory materials for this purpose. All students must have read the recommended literature—which should be doable in a few hours—and the introduction of the patient case and have prepared the first few questions for that case, until the stage where new patient information must be provided to proceed with the case.

Across the course, at each session three different students serve as a *peer teacher*, so all students have turns in this role. These peer teachers are provided with more information about the patient case and are therefore able to guide the group through the case. Although a *consultant* (clinician teacher) is present, his or her role is really that of a true consultant: remaining at the background, responding to questions, and only interrupting to clarify things and help the group process.

The meeting starts by having one of the peer teachers read the initial patient vignette out loud, introducing the patient and his or her complaint. After this, the first question is introduced. Students are randomly asked by peer teachers to give and substantiate answers. The peer teachers collect all answers. They monitor that all answers are given in a way that stimulates the group discussion. If necessary, they can provide hints based on their thorough preparation.

During the sessions, the peer teachers guide these discussions, as they provide handouts containing additional information about the patient. Usually one mini lecture (5 to maximum 10 min) is given by one of the peer teachers, summarizing an essential feature of the case, often a pathophysiological mechanism or background information about diagnostic tests.

At the end of the session, one of the non-peer teaching students, usually randomly chosen, is asked to summarize the case in 2–3 min, in a way that resembles case summaries for handovers in the clinical setting.

Participant Roles

All students should be made familiar with the rules before the start of the first CBCR session. An introductory session to set the stage is useful for that purpose.

The Student Role

It is essential that the students have read about the topic in advance and have prepared the first few general questions of the case. They do not know how the case will unfold, as they have limited information about the patient. They must therefore read about the major complaint of the patient to have enough background information.

Students should realize that this education requires verbally active participation. Verbalization of thoughts is essential in the acquisition of clinical reasoning skill, even if those thoughts later become more routine, encapsulated, and tacit (Schmidt and Boshuizen 1993).

Table 6.1 Typical table to be filled out during a CBCR session justifying how signs and symptoms confirm or disclaim particular hypotheses

[Fill in each cell: +; =; or −]	Hypotheses			
	1:…	2:…	3:…	4:…
[History finding 1]				
[History finding 2]				
[History finding 3]				
[Physical examination finding 1]				
[Physical examination finding 2]				

The Peer Teacher Role

Peer teachers perform an essential role in CBCR sessions since they act as teachers. Students have this role 2–3 times in a year and must prepare well for it.

The peer teachers must figure out in advance what pathology the patient has, guided by hints provided in their version of the case description. During the session, they should provide similar hints to students if needed and lead them through the case.

During the session the peer teachers are responsible for the active participation of all students in an equal manner. So they might give turns to students and proactively address the more silent students. They collect answers to case questions by summarizing items on a flip chart or board and letting students explain why they think the way they do. They are instructed to use tables to create a clear overview of answers given. See Table 6.1 for an example.

The three peer teacher students may distribute preparatory tasks among themselves before the session and during the session. One peer teacher can act as a chairperson for a series of questions, while one other can provide extra information or hints, and the third peer teacher summarizes after each question or discussion if needed. During the session, the peer teachers should regularly switch these sub-roles. All should be prepared to take all roles.

The Consultant Role

The consultant oversees the CBCR session, keeps a record of attendance, globally assesses the students' active participation, and provides feedback to students and peer teachers. He or she distributes peer teacher versions of written materials for a next session and completes evaluation forms.

Their most important role is guiding the CBCR sessions in an adaptive way, depending on the quality of the guidance already provided by peer teachers. This is very different from what many teachers are familiar with in traditional curricula, in which they are the primary source of information and have strong instructional tasks. It also differs from many other tutorial teaching formats where the teacher remains a central instructor deciding how to proceed. Problem-based learning arrangements come closest to demanding a similar teacher role (Barrows and Tamblyn 1980), but that role is not particularly clinically focused and does not require clinical experience as in CBCR education. CBCR is different. Peer teachers lead sessions and discussions, and the consultant only supports and helps when things are unclear, by asking clarifying questions or by offering perspectives when students think of rare and exotic diseases and forget or are unaware of the predominant epidemiology. Consultants usually stimulate peer teachers best to lead the group when they remain aside and only interfere when really necessary. This gives students a great responsibility and stimulates clinical thinking. If necessary of course, they can be consulted and give answers to questions from the group.

In most CBCR courses, the consultant keeps an attendance list for each session to register when students are present or absent. The course director receives these lists regularly and will have an overview of the attendance of every student.

Students should be evaluated on their preparation and active participation during the session in the clinical thinking of the group. The marks together can be part of the final grade. Consultants learning the dynamics of their group can develop a balanced impression of the participation of its members over sessions, which helps both the decision when to interrupt discussions to redirect the group if needed and how to score the students' participation.

After each session three new peer teachers receive the peer teachers' version of the next case to prepare for the next class. With a class of 12, nine sessions and three peer teachers per session, every student has this role once in four sessions. This way every student fulfills at least twice the role of peer teacher. The consultant coordinates this and ensures that each student regularly fulfills peer teacher tasks and he or she controls the distribution of peer teacher versions of the materials. The first peer teachers receive their version in or after the introductory session, at which meeting also the procedures of CBCR are explained.

As part of a continuous quality assurance of the course, it is very useful if consultants write down feedback about cases during or directly after sessions, such as linguistic errors, medical inadequacies or pedagogical improvements, and provide these comments to the CBCR course director.

CBCR Course Management

To organize a CBCR course in the curriculum, a course director or course manager needs to be appointed, as should be the case for any course. Tasks of the course director are planning sessions, preparing and delivering materials to consultants and students, collecting records of attendance and case evaluations, instructing students and faculty (consultants), serving as a contact person for students and consultants, evaluating and updating materials annually, and preparing and administering exams. At UMC Utrecht, the course management is carried out by a team of three and, in total, requires about a 0.2 full-time equivalent for 24 groups, i.e., 300 students, to be served.

The course director should make sure that there are no scheduling conflicts with other courses or exams. It is recommended to randomly assign students to groups. This improves group dynamics, allows struggling students to learn from others, and also challenges clever students to improve their argumentation by explaining their thoughts to their peers. During the course, the group should keep the same composition.

The course director should ensure that all consultants and students receive their respective versions of the course materials and should avoid that consultant versions are seen by students, as that may interfere with the desired reasoning process during the class. Consultants receive, in addition, peer teacher materials, forms for registration of attendance and for marking of students, and program evaluation forms. At UMC Utrecht a photograph of the students of each group is taken during the first session with students holding their names on a piece of paper. This helps consultants to know their students by face from the very start. The consultant keeps an overview of which students have been peer teachers and makes sure that all students perform their respective roles.

A general CBCR study guide should also be included in the folder for consultants. It contains the description of the course for the students and explains the rules and regulations of the course (see Chap. 10). For some CBCR cases, as a service for the consultant, additional literature can be included as well.

Recruiting and instructing consultants should be one of the course director's tasks. New consultants must become familiar with the course requirements and procedures. An annual faculty development workshop for new consultants is an excellent opportunity to supplement with oral instructions and discussions. More elaborate faculty development, as explained in Chap. 9, may include a volunteer student CBCR group meeting during such a workshop, with new consultants practicing or observing.

As is the case with new consultants, students are usually not familiar with CBCR before the course either. An annual information session, such as a lecture, is useful before the CBCR course starts and should elaborate on what the purposes and practice of CBCR are. Most practical aspects should be discussed, e.g., what is expected of students in their roles of regular students or peer teachers, what students should prepare for sessions, how sessions proceed, and what the end-of-term examination will look like. Tasks of students and peer teachers should be explained, but also the task of the consultant and the different setup of CBCR compared to other courses. It should be made clear that students are largely responsible for the CBCR sessions and that a good preparation of their part is essential to make sessions a success.

The CBCR course director oversees the cases written. All cases and case revisions should however be written or at least thoroughly checked by a specialist on the topic and preferably by someone who checks language, following instructions as elaborated in Chap. 8.

The course director should also be the responsible examiner, who designs and administers exams and analyzes and communicates results, if needed assisted by content experts. We refer for details to Chap. 7.

A CBCR Course Version Using Senior Medical Students as Consultants

In the most recent years at UMC Utrecht, the CBCR course uses final year medical students as consultants for second year medical students. This *near-peer* consultant role, with a 4-year difference in education, has proven to be a successful adaptation. All final year medical students at Utrecht have a 1-week mandatory teacher training course with different components (Zijdenbos et al. 2011). One component is a true teaching experience with second year medical students in at least one CBCR session. These near-peer consultants receive a thorough pedagogical instruction and receive the consultant version of the case materials for their session (Zijdenbos et al. 2010). The teacher training course is delivered in groups of 15 students who are prepared and debriefed before and after the CBCR session. Their role as a consultant includes facilitating, evaluating, and scoring students and peer teachers for active participation. Across the year all ±300 final year students must practice this teaching, usually in a team of two, once or twice with one of the 24 groups in one of their nine sessions. The schedules are organized in a way to provide all second year groups with near-peer consultants. Both the sixth year students and the second year students show consistent favorable evaluations of their experiences as receivers and providers of clinical reasoning training, since the start of this model in 2006 (Zijdenbos et al. 2010).

Evidence of Effectiveness

As said, CBCR courses have been well received across decades of implementation. Student ratings are usually high. There is no doubt that students and schools consider the courses valuable. A comparative study to objectify this impression has not been carried out however. The reason is that this curriculum model has been applied across complete cohorts and because the course did not replace a different course with similar objectives, which excludes a suitable comparison group. In other words, there is no treatment comparison with the same or similar students possible. Comparing the effects of curricula with and without the CBCR course is difficult because of methodological and confounding problems. However, one interesting curriculum comparison study has been reported in the literature. In 1996 Schmidt et al. reported superior performance of an Amsterdam cohort of students that compared two other universities in the preclinical years 2 and 3 (Schmidt et al. 1996).

The Amsterdam curriculum had recently introduced a CBCR course that later stood model for the Utrecht CBCR course (ten Cate 1994). The effect that Schmidt et al. found may have been caused by the CBCR course in that curriculum. While this is speculation, no other explanation has been offered for the superiority of the Amsterdam curriculum in the preclinical years of a measure of clinical reasoning.

Finally, the development of illness scripts, an objective of the CBCR course by students, was recently studied and found to be better in preclinical students for cases discussed in the CBCR course than other common cases not studied in the CBCR course (Keemink et al. n.d.).

References

Barrows, H. S., & Tamblyn, R. M. (1980). *Problem-based learning. An approach to medical education*. New York: Springer.
Keemink, Y. et al. (n.d.) Illness script development through Case-Based Clinical Reasoning training. *Submitted*.
Schmidt, H. G., & Boshuizen, H. P. A. (1993). On acquiring expertise in medicine. *Educational Psychology Review, 5*(3), 205–221.
Schmidt, H., et al. (1996). The development of diagnostic competence: Comparison of a problem-based, and integrated and a conventional medical curriculum. *Academic Medicine, 71*(6), 658–664.
ten Cate, O. (1994). Training case-based clinical reasoning in small groups [Dutch]. *Nederlands Tijdschrift voor Geneeskunde, 138*, 1238–1243.
Zijdenbos, I. L., et al. (2010). A student-led course in clinical reasoning in the core curriculum. *International Journal of Medical Education, 1*, 42–46.
Zijdenbos, I., Fick, T., & ten Cate, O. (2011). How we offer all medical students training in basic teaching skills. *Medical Teacher, 33*(1), 24–26.

Open Access This chapter is licensed under the terms of the Creative Commons Attribution 4.0 International License (http://creativecommons.org/licenses/by/4.0/), which permits use, sharing, adaptation, distribution and reproduction in any medium or format, as long as you give appropriate credit to the original author(s) and the source, provide a link to the Creative Commons license and indicate if changes were made.

The images or other third party material in this chapter are included in the chapter's Creative Commons license, unless indicated otherwise in a credit line to the material. If material is not included in the chapter's Creative Commons license and your intended use is not permitted by statutory regulation or exceeds the permitted use, you will need to obtain permission directly from the copyright holder.

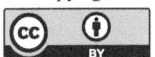

Chapter 7
Assessment of Clinical Reasoning Using the CBCR Test

Olle ten Cate

A CBCR course for preclinical students should be completed with some form of student evaluation, as any course in a medical curriculum should be concluded with a valid decision about the extent to which every student has reached the objectives of the course. Many students proceed through education with one predominant, returning question in mind: *what must I do to pass this course and its examination?* This guides their efforts in learning, and as the saying goes, "assessment drives learning" or "students rather learn what you *inspect* than what you *expect*." This is not something to be disappointed about, but a fact of university life that should be understood and respected. After all, it is the school that sets these rules. However, the lesson to be learned is that assessment should be aligned with the educational objectives in such way that what we inspect is exactly what we expect (Biggs 1996). If we test students on clinical reasoning skills, the examination should rather not consist of four-item multiple-choice or true/false questions that focus on factual knowledge. That would drive students in the direction of rehearsing the systems approach to biomedical knowledge that, as we have shown, is in contrast with the patient-oriented approach in CBCR sessions. Assessment needs to focus more specifically on clinical reasoning skill, acknowledging however the importance of biomedical knowledge for clinical reasoning. That should include questions like: What, at this stage, is a likely differential diagnosis? What findings would you expect to find with physical examination if hypothesis X were true? Which laboratory tests of the ordering list would you check for this patient at this stage? In other words, multiple options from a larger array of possibilities can suit the assessment of clinical reasoning better than standard four-option MC questions.

O. ten Cate (✉)
Center for Research and Development of Education, University Medical Center Utrecht, Utrecht, The Netherlands
e-mail: T.J.tenCate@umcutrecht.nl

The CBCR Test as Developed at the University Medical Center Utrecht

In 2010 a specific written assessment format was developed for the CBCR course at the University Center Utrecht, which has been in place ever since that time. The aim of the design was to align the test as closely as possible with both the CBCR course as delivered and the desired future skill of patient-oriented clinical reasoning.

The case-based questions all follow the course of the clinical encounter, starting with a case title that reflects the initial information the physician normally would have (age, gender, and main complaint) and a short clinical presentation vignette. Then, a series of questions about the case unfolds.

Features from different established item types as discussed in Chap. 5 have been incorporated:

- Relatively long lists of options, such as used in *extended matching* questions and long menu items
- A differential diagnostic approach from the *comprehensive integrated puzzle* items through the "alternative scenarios" approach
- The addition of new information to alter a hypothesis as used in the *script concordance test*.

The first and foremost feature of the Utrecht CBCR test is the integrated, patient-oriented nature of the test. The unit of focus is a patient with several option lists (diagnostic hypotheses, history findings, physical examination findings, diagnostic findings, management options, etc.) that all pertain to focused questions following from the initial patient presentation or from follow-up information about this patient. The test has a limited number of cases but a broad enough set to reduce the threat of case specificity and has a series of questions within each case. The CBCR test has the following characteristics.

Alignment with Actual Cases Discussed

An important purpose of the CBCR course for junior students is to mentally "install" a basic framework of a limited number of illness scripts. The Utrecht CBCR test therefore closely follows the cases discussed during the CBCR sessions. There is no expectation of substantial *transfer of learning*, i.e., of a benefit of studying cases for the ability to handle other cases and no aim to test that transfer ability early in the medical curriculum. Indeed, an additional aim of closely following the cases studied is to reinforce the learned scripts both by rehearsing for the test and during the test itself. For senior medical students, who have acquired a basic mental framework of illness scripts in their long-term memory, it may well be recommended to deviate from cases discussed, to gradually test a more general clinical reasoning ability, but this is not the aim of the end-of-course CBCR test for the preclinical students.

Cases, Options Lists, and Scenarios

The case is the unit of focus for test items. The question starts with a short case vignette that usually resembles an initial presentation of the patient at the primary care doctor's office, the emergency department, or elsewhere, similar to the start of a CBCR education case. Several option lists that may vary in length from 5 to 25 or more options accompany the case presentation. These lists include the following nine optional categories: (a) diagnoses, (b) history questions, (c) history findings, (d) physical examination procedures, (e) physical examination findings, (f) diagnostic test options, (g) diagnostic test findings, (h) management options, and (i) prognosis. Usually, a limited number of lists (4 or 5) will be used for one case. The distinction between history questions and history findings is that either the question can be "What are the [two] most relevant next questions to ask?" or "Which [three] history findings would you expect if hypothesis X were true?" (or equivalent questions). This also holds for physical examination and diagnostic tests. All questions may ask to check as many options from a list as the item writer finds suitable, e.g., "Which four lab findings would you expect to find given what you know about this patient?" However, the number of correct options should not be more than one third of the total list, and preferably much less, to avoid successful guessing.

Questions may be about a differential diagnosis following from the initial case vignette, but cases generally include one or more sequential *scenarios*. A scenario is defined as a deviation from the initial course of happenings or findings, but still relates to the same patient (age, sex, main complaint, and initial vignette). A scenario usually starts like this. "Scenario B. Presume, the radiology of this patient's thorax shows a lump in the left lower lung, which two hypotheses from the list (a) Diagnoses would now be most likely?" Or "Scenario C. Presume, the radiology of this patient's thorax would show no pathology, which two hypotheses from the list (a) Diagnoses would now be most likely?" Case title, initial vignette, and all options lists are identical throughout a case, but correct options (and the number of requested options) vary.

In practice, most cases include one to three scenarios. When there is only one scenario, the word *scenario* is not used.

CBCR Test Quality Findings Since 2010

Between December 2010 and April 2017, the test has been administered 14 times, with on average about 12 cases and 50 items (about four items per case), for cohorts of about 300 students. The test reliability averaged 0.73 (Cronbach's alpha) for tests with an average duration of not much more than 1 h. In this course, spread across 8 months, a test is administered twice (in December and April), and the final score combines both sub-scores. This combined score would compare with a test with 24 cases, 2–2.5 h of testing and an estimated average reliability of 0.84 (estimated with the Spearman-Brown formula). This is more than satisfactory and more efficient than key feature tests (Page and Bordage 1995).

The test questions were derived from small group CBCR cases, supplemented with cases presented in a lecture hall. We will not expand on the latter cases, which constituted a minority of the items, but they were suitable for a similar approach to clinical reasoning testing, given the large group education format (Borleffs et al. 2003). Given the richness of the cases discussed in het CBCR sessions, it was possible to devise new questions for each test, hardly without using any previous questions.

Electronic and Paper Versions

All CBCR tests except one were administered electronically. The first version of the test was not much more than a protected interface. After logging in with a general password, candidates could access all questions per case on one screen: The left side of the screen showed a series of questions and open fill-in-the-blank-slots; on the right side of the screen, all relevant options lists were displayed. Candidates were then asked to enter a three-digit number into the relevant slots at the left side of the screen. The resulting file was exported as an Excel® file, available after the test administration and suitable for analysis with an elaborate Excel® analysis application and statistical software.

A next version of the application showed a professional interface with check boxes instead of fill-in-the-blank slots. Currently, a commercial test administration firm, TestVision® (www.testvision.nl), has incorporated the CBCR item format requirements into a professional application.

What the Utrecht CBCR Test Does Not Provide

The Utrecht CBCR test approach has limitations. In clinical reasoning, a logical question is "what is the most likely diagnosis?". All question types that are not constructed response suffer from some cueing, as the answer can be chosen from a list. Script concordance testing and the comprehensive integrative puzzle approaches have simply given up on this requirement as diagnostic hypotheses are given and not asked (Charlin et al. 2000; Ber 2003; Groothoff et al. 2008). CBCR test questions provide a list to choose from that can be as long as the item writer wishes, thereby somewhat limiting this cueing, similar to extended matching questions and long menu questions (Case and Swanson 1998; Schuwirth et al. 1996). The recommended length is 20 options. In practice, they are often shorter and sometimes longer.

Another feature that is not supported is the possibility to evaluate a chain of interdependent reasoning questions and answers of a candidate, requiring conditional links between consecutive answers (*if the student chooses X on item 1, then item 2 will be adapted*). That possibility is not provided. It would be possible to value an answer differently if it follows upon a previous *wrong* answer, as the two answers may be correctly related to each other. If the chain of reasoning becomes longer, however, the potential branches to be evaluated would quickly become too many to manage. The use of parallel scenarios however compensates this by the possibility of branching options from the same patient. A question of a parallel scenario always starts with "Presume,.." e.g., "Presume, you have received result X from diagnostic test Y, what then would be the most likely diagnosis?".

Finally, the current use of CBCR test methodology does not allow for weighing of items within answers ("Provide a differential diagnosis of three in a correct order of likelihood"); that now requires multiple questions ("What is the most likely diagnosis?" and "Name two other diagnostic hypotheses"). These are technical limitations that in the future may be solved with sophisticated software.

Rules and Regulations Around the Utrecht CBCR Test

In practice, the Utrecht CBCR test is administered twice a year, each for half of the final score. Students pass the course requirements if their final test score, combined with proof of active participation in the course as a student and as a peer teacher, if satisfactory. As participation also yields a score, test and participation scores are combined to cover 88% and 12% of the final score, respectively, which was found to be a useful ratio. We will not expand on how the participation rate per student is calculated, but details can be found in the model study guide in Chap. 10. Students who do not pass the requirements can opt for a retake of the examination.

Issues of Validity of the CBCR Test

The Utrecht CBCR tests as applied since 2010 have an undisputed content validity, as they are built upon cases that are used in the course, and they cover all cases.

The construct validity of the Utrecht CBCR test approach remains to be investigated.

Example

Table 7.1 shows an example of a CBCR test question, derived from a case that is used in education. The representation of the question may have different forms when presented as an actual test. The initial case vignette should remain visible while students proceed with scenarios through the case. Supplementary visual information, such as a photo of the patient, an X-ray image, or others may appear when indicated.

Table 7.1 Example of a CBCR case translated to test questions

---

Case 1. A 36-year old woman with headache
A 36-year old female patient presents at her family doctor with a severe headache.

Case 1, Scenario A
The patient has a diffuse, clamping headache, occurring frequently in the last month. Last year she had similar complaints when she was very busy at work. On physical examination you find no abnormalities.

1. Which diagnosis is most likely? Choose 1 option from 'diagnoses'
2. Which diagnostic test option is now indicated? Choose 1 option from 'diagnostic test options'.
3. Which management options are now suitable? Choose 3 options from 'management options'.

Case 1, Scenario B
Presume, that the patient had experienced several episodes of severe headache during the past two months. In the past she has had similar complaints. There is no fever.

4. One of the diagnoses you consider is migraine. Which history features would you expect to find if this diagnosis is true? Choose 5 options from 'history features'

Presume, you are thinking of a cluster headache.
5. Which findings during physical examination make this diagnosis more likely? Choose 2 options from 'physical examination'.

Case 1, Scenario C
Based on the history and physical examination you consider temporal arteritis and cluster headache.
6. Which diagnostic test options can help to distinguish between them? Choose 2 options from 'diagnostic test options'.

Diagnoses	History findings
Acute glaucoma	Alcohol provokes the complaints
Alcohol hangover	Duration: 1 to 2 days
Analgesics headache	Duration: several minutes
Cerebral tumor	Duration: several weeks
Cluster headache	First epileptic attack 1 week ago
Dentogenic headache	Menstruation provokes the complaints
Encephalitis	Morning vomiting
Hypoglycemia	Pain depends on position
Influenza	Pain is bilateral
Meningitis	Pain is clamping
Migraine	Pain is throbbing
Posttraumatic headache	Pain is unilateral
Pre-eclampsia	Pain started acute
Refraction abnormalities	Patient has dental problems
Sinusitis	Patient is 8 months pregnant
Subarachnoid hemorrhage	Patient is 8 weeks pregnant
Subdural or epidural hematoma	Patient is hypersensitive to light and noise
Temporal arteritis	Patient is nauseous and vomits
Tension headache	Patient sees flashes of light
Trigl neuralgiaemina	Patient uses painkillers in high doses
	Recent personality change

Physical examination findings	Diagnostic test options
Decreased visual acuity	Biopsy temporal artery
Fever	Cell count and differentiation
Increased blood pressure	CT-angiography
Increased tear production	CT-scan or MRI-scan
Miosis (pupillary constriction)	EEG
Neck stiffness	ESR
Neurological impairment	No diagnostic tests
Pain on palpation of temporal artery	Rontgen photo neck/skull
Reduced level of consciousness	

Management options	
Discuss measures to achieve stress reduction	
Headache diary	
Refer to specialist	
Send for emergency treatment	
Strong painkillers (opioids)	
Watchful waiting, unless complaints worsen	

Scoring of Items

Once students have taken the test, a file results with all answers. A common format is an Excel® file with rows per student and columns of answers per option. See Fig. 7.1
for an example. The unit of scoring is the option. If Question 1 from Case 1, Scenario A, asks for a differential diagnosis of four hypotheses that need to be considered with this patient, all students will have an answer for a, b, c, d. Scores are counted for each question into a sum score of 0 to 4 or 5, depending on the number of options requested in that question. For psychometric purposes (calculation of Cronbach's alpha reliability and item analysis) the unit of analysis is the question (but there are arguments to use scenarios or cases as units of analysis). As with any test, we recommend to conduct an item analysis to determine whether any items need to be removed before final scores for students are disclosed. Those final scores can be calculated in different ways. The Utrecht procedure is to first calculate the mean guessing rate per item (e.g. 20 or 25%) and take that percentage of the maximum score as a bottom score. E.g., a test of 50 questions and 120 options, with an average guessing score of 21% yields a bottom score of 25. Subtracting that from the maximum score of 120 means that all students receive a score between 0 and 95 points. As we want to end the CBCR course with a final score that combines two test scores (88%) and a score for participation (12%), and because we use a 100-point scale, each test score must be recalculated to a 0-44 points range.

Case	Case 1														Case 2								
Scenario	Case 1 – Scenario A						Case 1 – Scen. B								Case 2 – Scen. A				Case 2 – Scen. B				
Question	1				2		3	4				5			6			7	8	9	10			
Option	a	b	c	d	a	b	a	a	b	c	d	a	b	c	a	b	c	a	a	a	b	a	b	c	d
Student 1																									
Student 2																									
Student 3																									
Et cetera																									

Fig. 7.1 Possible data format for analysis

Checklist for Item Writers

We end with a checklist for writers of test questions for CBCR-tests. Box 7.1 includes a number of pitfalls to avoid and recommendations to follow.

> **Box 7.1 Checklist for Item Writers of the Utrecht CBCR Test**
> 1. Always include *age*, *sex* and *main complaint*, and *sign or symptom* in the case title.
> 2. Always relate to *this* individual patient. Instead of "Which two physical examination findings do patients with complaint X always have," ask: "Which two physical examination features do you expect to find when examining this patient, based on her complaint X?". Stimulate students to think from a patient-oriented perspective, also during the test. "...do you expect to find..." is the aimed typical hypothesis-driven thinking mode and is regularly used in CBCR test items. In many cases, it is sensible to add "...if this hypothesis is correct." Check whether an answer requires a preceding case vignette; if not, it is probably not a question about the individual patient.
> 3. When writing items, stay close to how the information arrived at the physician, e.g., the history as the patient presents its physical examination as what the physicians sees or hears), rather that interpreting and summarizing with semantic qualifiers (avoid "The patient provides a family history of cardiovascular disease," and rather "...has yellow sclerae" than "...is icteric"), unless the presentation would be a discharge letter from a hospital.
> 4. Be specific about the number of requested options from the list (and avoid "at least" or "maximum number" of options to be checked).
> 5. Make sure that the list contains options that do not overlap or include each other. Also, do not include two items in the list that evidently exclude each other, while the list contains other options ("age younger than 30, age 30 or older, and age 50" should not all be used in one listing).
> 6. Formulate finding options specific rather than general (*Age 46* rather than *older than 40*; "Pain since three weeks" rather than "Pain since quite some time"); again formulate how this information is presented by the patient.
> 7. Intersperse questions with small follow-up information text. *The following lab results are reported: [...]*; then continue with a next question.
> 8. Start a new *scenario* if there is a deviation from earlier information or questions. The first question of a new scenario typically starts with "Scenario B. Presume, the patient had said/shown/...." If there is no branching or deviation from earlier information, "scenario" terminology is not needed. Students must understand the significance of the "scenario" terminology in their instruction about this test.

(continued)

Box 7.1 (continued)

9. Avoid linking a question to a previous question (e.g., "What are the two best management options for this diagnosis" after the question "What is the most likely diagnosis") as this requires sophisticated analysis technology, unless the questions are scored by hand. The solution is to start with "Presume, the diagnosis X has been confirmed, what would then be..." Make sure that this diagnosis does not disclose the previous answer, e.g., by choosing as X something that is *not* the most likely diagnosis. Likewise, do not use the option lists *history questions*, *physical examination procedures*, and *diagnostic test options* in such way that a follow-up text or scenario reveals the answer to a previous question.
10. Try to find an adequate representation of questions across cases and an adequate balance of questions about history, physical examination, diagnostic tests, and management.
11. Make sure a CBCR test question is always reviewed by a colleague *without the model answer* before it is accepted. One reason is that option lists may include more items that must be considered correct than initially anticipated. A recommendation is to ask a few senior students to take the draft test. That should reveal most major flaws.

References

Ber, R. (2003). The CIP (comprehensive integrative puzzle) assessment method. *Medical Teacher, 25*(2), 171–176.

Biggs, J. (1996). Enhancing teaching through constructive alignment. *Higher Education, 32*, 347–364.

Borleffs, J. C. C., et al. (2003). "Clinical reasoning theater": A new approach to clinical reasoning education. *Academic Medicine: Journal of the Association of American Medical Colleges, 78*(3), 322–325.

Case, S. M., & Swanson, D. B. (1998). *Constructing written test questions for the basic and clinical sciences* (2nd ed.). Philadelphia: National Board of Medical Examiners.

Charlin, B., et al. (2000). The script concordance test: A tool to assess the reflective clinician. *Teaching and learning in medicine, 12*(4), 189–195.

Groothoff, J. W., et al. (2008). Growth of analytical thinking skills over time as measured with the MATCH test. *Medical Education, 42*(10), 1037–1043.

Page, G., & Bordage, G. (1995). The Medical Council of Canada's key features project: A more valid written examination of clinical decision-making skills. *Academic Medicine, 70*(2), 104–110.

Schuwirth, L. W., et al. (1996). Computerized long-menu questions as an alternative to open-ended questions in computerized assessment. *Medical Education, 30*(1), 50–55.

Open Access This chapter is licensed under the terms of the Creative Commons Attribution 4.0 International License (http://creativecommons.org/licenses/by/4.0/), which permits use, sharing, adaptation, distribution and reproduction in any medium or format, as long as you give appropriate credit to the original author(s) and the source, provide a link to the Creative Commons license and indicate if changes were made.

The images or other third party material in this chapter are included in the chapter's Creative Commons license, unless indicated otherwise in a credit line to the material. If material is not included in the chapter's Creative Commons license and your intended use is not permitted by statutory regulation or exceeds the permitted use, you will need to obtain permission directly from the copyright holder.

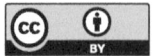

Chapter 8
Writing CBCR Cases

Olle ten Cate and Maria van Loon

Case-based teaching is considered a superior method of teaching for a variety of professional domains. Its success depends both on the way education is enhanced by adequate facilitation by teacher and on the quality of cases used (Kim et al. 2006). Dolmans et al. and Kim and colleagues have provided guidelines for effective case writing in health professions education (Dolmans et al. 1997; Kim et al. 2006). Working with adequate cases in problem-based learning is considered to stir situational interest in students during education, more than direct instruction (Schmidt et al. 2011). In a broad literature review, Kim and co-workers conclude that written clinical cases are most effective if they show five core attributes (Kim et al. 2006). They should be:

(a) Relevant (adjusted to the level of the learner, aligned with goals and objectives, and with an adequate setting of the case narrative)
(b) Realistic (showing authenticity, including distractors, providing a gradual disclosure of content)
(c) Engaging (providing a rich content with multiple perspectives and with branching of content)
(d) Challenging (sufficiently difficult, being new or atypical cases for the level of the learner, with adequate case structure, and including multiple cases)
(e) Instructional (building upon prior knowledge, incorporating feedback, and using educational or didactic aids where possible and adequately assessed).

O. ten Cate (✉)
Center for Research and Development of Education, University Medical Center Utrecht, Utrecht, The Netherlands
e-mail: T.J.tenCate@umcutrecht.nl

M. van Loon
University Medical Center Utrecht, Utrecht, The Netherlands
e-mail: mariavloon@gmail.com

CBCR cases should meet most, if not all, of these conditions. The authors provide 21 more detailed distinct and useful recommendations. There is one exception. While the authors recommend using atypical cases, in CBCR training for preclinical students, with a focus on establishing core illness scripts, we believe that atypical cases should be avoided.

The choice of cases for CBCR courses is determined by the objectives of intended illness scripts to be acquired and internalized by preclinical students. They should cover important medical conditions that serve as a strong clinical knowledge foundation, even in its inherent limitations at this stage of training, for students before they start with clinical clerkships. Writing cases for CBCR sessions must be done by clinicians with practice experience in the theme of the case, but may be edited by experienced CBCR consultants or CBCR course developers. This chapter explains how to write CBCR cases.

Overview

CBCR cases consist of an introductory text describing a patient case in the way it is presented to a clinician. As a variant, two cases with similar presentations but different diagnoses within a differential may be worked through in one session. Alternatively, one case can be spread over two sessions, although that rarely happens. The start of the case may be at a primary care doctor's office, at an emergency department, at an outpatient clinic, or on the clinical ward after referral. The case description, after the initial vignette, continues with questions and assignments, at fixed moments with the provision of findings from further history, supplementary physical examination, or diagnostic investigations, distributed and read out loud by peer teachers during the session at the right moment. A full case includes the complete course of a problem from the initial presentation to follow up after treatment. Often, cases concentrate on key stages of this course. Case descriptions should refer to relevant (patho-)physiological backgrounds and basic sciences such as anatomy, biochemistry, cell biology, and physiology and whenever relevant during the case.

Three Versions of the Written Case

Each CBCR case is not only a *student version* and a teacher (*consultant*) *version* but also an in-between-type *peer teacher version*. As CBCR sessions are led by two or three peer teachers who need to be instructed how to guide the meeting, they are not provided with comprehensive answers and solutions to questions, since they must practice clinical reasoning themselves as well. The consultant should have all answers available if needed.

Student Version

The student version includes general instructions, an initial case vignette, and several questions. The general instructions consist of the objectives for this case; the literature students should read when preparing for the session and instructions about which questions they need to answer before the session. The student version of the case is provided to all students, including the peer teachers.

Peer Teacher Version

The peer teacher version contains the student version information but is more extended. Only the peer teachers for a particular session receive the peer teachers' version through the consultant of the group. They should not share this information with other students before the session.

The peer teacher version provides hints and instructions with every question. These guide them toward the correct answer without directly disclosing answers or diagnoses. Any instructions given for a question suggest the peer teachers how to deal with this question: to use a table or PowerPoint®, to use a role-play, or to use instructions on how to stimulate students to come with proper arguments. Peer teachers also receive handouts, i.e., additional information about the patient on history findings, physical examination findings, diagnostic test results, and management policy, each to be disclosed during the meeting at the right moment. Finally, most cases include a peer teacher assignment for a mini-lecture (5 to a maximum of 10 min) about a relevant pathophysiological topic or background information about diagnostic tests.

Consultant Version

The full consultant version of the CBCR case includes all information, suggestions, and hints for peer teachers and all answers in detail for all questions, as much as is necessary for a non-expert clinician, and includes all patient information that peer teachers should disclose during the session.

Selecting Themes for CBCR Cases

When selecting cases to be included in the CBCR course, it is useful to take the following points into consideration:

- Cases should deal with important, i.e., common medical problems that represent illness scripts that all students will need to have in mind when they embark on clinical clerkships.
- In addition, uncommon problems may be included when the problems represent severe conditions that should be treated, i.e., that should never be missed.
- Cases should have educational value. They should include enough 'meat' to make an instructive session, preferably both clinically and in the field of the applied basic sciences.
- Cases should preferably represent various clinical domains and make students aware that clinical reasoning is applicable in every specialty.
- Cases that are interesting primarily from an ethical or communicative perspective may be less apt for CBCR, which must train students in clinical reasoning rather than get them acquainted with non-medical or ethical problems.

Cases may be derived from actual patients and then be adapted for educational purposes. Cases can be written by primary care doctors or by specialists and should focus on complaints from different domains. Medical specialist writers should be aware that most cases start when a patient visits a primary care doctor for the first time with an undifferentiated condition often not confined to one specialty. When writing a case, the complaint of the patient needs to be the central point of focus.

Common complaints (e.g. 'headache') may eventually turn out to be a less common diagnosis that, however, should never be missed (e.g. 'meningitis'). The aim of clinical reasoning is taking various causal options into account. Cases can branch off in alternative scenarios ('now suppose the lab results had shown no signs of an infection, what then would have been your hypothesis?'). The development of illness scripts in the student's mind should eventually represent a network of related disease patterns with interlinks. That is why discussions about differential diagnoses and the use of alternative scenarios within a case are important.

CBCR courses can be conducted in several curriculum years. The complexity of the cases should therefore depend on the developmental level of the students. During the first year, students are not yet familiar with illness scripts; the students will not yet be aware of making a differential diagnosis and how to take a medical history. CBCR in the first year of medical school is possible but should deal with simple cases, and the reasoning process may take quite some time. The complexity of the case should increase over the years, and the time allocated to work through a case should decrease. More advanced student groups may handle two or more cases in a session or a case with several scenarios branching off. Still, independent of year and level of the student, a CBCR case always reflects an entire patient case from the moment that the patient enters the doctor's office until the moment that a plan has been made for management.

An Annotated Template for CBCR Cases

The following section of this chapter represents a template to write cases. We recommend following a standard template. Students should not be distracted by unnecessary variations in the format of case descriptions over a course, unless the content dictates so. It is therefore recommended to stick with one format across all cases. The format below has been proven useful for many years at UMC Utrecht. Before a series of cases are written, it is advisable to start copying this template (without the annotations between brackets), adapted if necessary, and then use it for all cases.

> **All bold-face text is to be used for paragraph headings**
> [Annotations and explanations are given between brackets]
> This framework is an example. Cases may deviate from this framework, depending on the content of the case, on the insights of the case writer and for educational reasons.

*****

Title: A ... year old ... with ....

[A CBCR title typically is the shortest summary of the patient presentation and always includes *age*, *gender* and *main complaint or problem*. A title should not be 'Shortness of breath', but it could be 'A 23-year old man with sudden shortness of breath'.]

Introduction and Objective
[An introduction for the case may be given. However, it should not disclose essential information that must be sorted out by the students during the case elaboration. This also holds for the objectives of the session. What may be stated in the introduction is the frequency or epidemiology of the type of problem with which this patient presents.]

Preparation
Students need to prepare questions ... - ... at home.
 [State here what students should prepare for this session from both preparatory reading and answering of questions. Literature may also refer to previous courses or specific references, websites, etc. Students have less literature to read for preparation than peer teachers. On average, student preparation time for a case is 2 h and for peer teachers 4 h. It is not useful to ask students to spend days preparing for a case – that will simply not happen, so limit the preparation to what is feasible.

All students need to answer some questions at home before the session. Typically these are all questions until the first additional patient information (handout) is provided by the peer teachers. Later questions may be speculatively answered.]

Assessment
[Assessment for participation should be clarified here.]

Suggested Time Schedule
[An estimation should be made of the suggested time per question during the 2 h meeting. This prevents spending too much time on the first question(s) and the need to rush for the last question(s).]

CBCR Case Stage I: Presentation of the Patient's Problem

Case
[This is where the actual case starts. A 'stage' is a period of time between two moments of provided patient information, so in between handouts. Stage I begins with an introductory text or vignette of, usually, 50–200 words, depicting the patient's initial story, question, complaint, or evident symptoms before history taking. This means that the information will only state that what the patient will tell the doctor directly, without having to ask for it. This section should stimulate the students to start thinking of additional history questions they want to ask the patient to gain more information. Stage I also introduces the doctor, referring to specialty, position, and location.

For example, '*You are a general practitioner. In your office, a 15 year old boy Victor, accompanied by his mother, presents in the morning with complaints of severe pain in the left leg, after a football match yesterday afternoon. Victor had a sleepless night, as his leg developed a reddish painful lump*'. Patient information should always be printed in italics.]

Question 1 State in your own words what the main problem seems to be

[This question may be phrased differently, but should typically reflect the first thoughts of the doctor; i.e. what diseases or major disease groups can you think of?]

Hints for peer teachers
[After each question, one or more hints for the peer teachers are given. These are not printed in the students' version, but are included in the consultant's version. These usually do not disclose the answer to the question, but help peer teachers to guide the group process. If questions are difficult, references may be given.

Peer teachers can get pedagogical instructions in the hints, e.g. that they should always first ask student-members of the group to answer the question and only then react to the given answers. It is important to realize that all students of the group must be stimulated to think along. Direct answers from the peer teachers or from the consultant often block students from active involvement].

Background information for the consultant
[After each question also 'background information for the consultant' is given. It includes the answer and sometimes variations of the answer to the question and explanatory details.

Remember that consultants are clinicians, but not necessarily a specialist on this particular subject. It is important to provide basic background information so they are able to help the students when they get stuck. References may be given, but information that is not instantly available may not help very much on the spot].

Question 2 Provide all hypotheses you have at this moment about the pathology and the cause of the signs and symptoms, grouped in three categories (I: likely, II: less likely, III: not very likely, but not excluded)

[Before history taking, physical examination, and investigations, the clinical reasoning is guided by hypotheses. This is a sample question to train students to develop hypotheses and, at the same time, to weight the likelihood of cases.]

Hints for peer teachers
[Peer teachers may be provided with general categories of causes, i.e. cardiovascular and metabolic.]

Background information for the consultant
[Consultants should get a list of hypotheses.]

Question 3 Which questions should be asked to discriminate between the most relevant hypotheses?

Hints for peer teachers
[Peer teachers should stimulate students to formulate questions in a way to ask it directly to the patient, i.e. *when do you experience this complaint?* Every student should think of at least two questions. A suggestion for the peer teachers could be to let one student think of a question and let his/her neighbour tell how this helps in differentiating between hypotheses.]

Background information for the consultant
[Consultants need to be provided with a list of the most common questions and how the answers can differentiate between several causes.]

Table 8.1 Hypotheses versus findings

	Hypotheses			
	Migraine	Cluster headache	[Hypothesis 3]	[Hypothesis 4]
Complaints since 2 weeks				
[History information b]				
[History information c]				
[History information d]				

Stage II: Results from History Taking Are Provided

Question 4   How does this information influence the differential diagnosis?

Hints for peer teachers

[Peer teachers should make sure that the information that is given in this handout was also asked for by the students during the previous question. If needed, the consultant can stimulate to do this.

Peer teachers should now be asked to draw a grid table on the blackboard or flip chart, as shown in Table 8.1.

This chart forces students think of why which questions are asked by the doctor.

Which information from history taking is important for which hypothesis?

A (+) should be added in the table when an answer pleas for a hypothesis. A (−) should be added if the answer pleas against a hypothesis, and a (+/−) should be added if an answer does not differentiate.]

Background information for the consultant

[Consultants should receive a full sample chart, filled out by the case writer.]

> **Handout 1**
> *(shown on the screen and read out loud)*
> [Peer teachers provide the results of the history taking. This information is printed on a handout or projected on a screen. If it is short, it may suffice to have peer teachers read the information. The handout text can then be provided at the end of the session together with other patient information. If the history information is very long, it may be helpful to provide a real handout at this stage during the session. A reading break is then necessary. In that case students also practice to filter the essential information from the handout.
>
> Peer teachers find the handouts in their CBCR case description. The information in the handout is written as a story, i.e. '*The headache started suddenly 2 weeks ago and the patient was forced to stay in bed with the lights of. She never experienced anything like this before. Etc…*'. A uniform layout for the patient information is printed in italics.]

8 Writing CBCR Cases

Question 5 Which parts of physical examination are required, in order to exclude some unlikely, but important hypotheses? Which examinations are necessary to confirm the most likely hypothesis and to discriminate between others?

Hints for peer teachers
[Students should be stimulated to argue specifically why they want to perform a certain examination. Peer teachers can write down for every remaining hypothesis what the students expect to find.]

Background information for the consultant
[Consultants should receive a full sample chart, filled out by the case writer.]

Stage III: Results from Physical Examination Are Provided

Handout 2
(shown on the screen and read out loud)
[Peer teachers read out loud the findings with physical examination, or, if necessary because of its length, hand out this information (text in italics). This could give a full picture of the physical findings (PE), or may just give a focussed result of the PE. Depending on the case, some new PE information may be provided later, if it appears to be necessary to complete the physical examination at a later stage. The information in the handout is written as a story.]

Question 6 Which hypotheses now remain as a differential diagnosis to be investigated further?

Hints for peer teachers
[Peer teachers may draw a similar table as with Question 4, or extend the table at the lower side to include the physical examination and then walk through all initial hypotheses and confirm which are left over to be considered.
A (+) should be added in the table when an answer pleas for a hypothesis. A (−) should be added if the answer pleas against a hypothesis, and a (+/−) should be added if an answer does not differentiate.]

Background information for the consultant
[Consultants receive the table with the results from the PE and how the results influence the remaining hypotheses.]

Question 7 Which Diagnostic Investigations Need to Be Done to Confirm or Exclude Remaining Diagnoses?

Hints for peer teachers

[Depending on the stage of the students in their curriculum, they may have much knowledge of diagnostic procedures or not. But even students with primarily basic science knowledge must be able to speculate on what is physically wrong and how one would learn to know what is the matter. Hints provided for the peer teachers may be, e.g. *think of specific haematological and/or radiological tests.*]

Background information for the consultant

[A list of answers is provided for the consultant. For non-common diagnostic tests, a brief overview of the expected results is given as well.]

Mini Lecture by One of the Peer Teachers

[This could be a good moment for a mini lecture. One of the peer teachers gives a short explanatory presentation (5 min) on aspects of pathology or pathophysiology as assigned by the case writer.

The goal of the mini lecture is to provide additional information for the students about the main complaint or certain group of diagnoses, diagnostic tests, or treatment. It should not, however, reveal the eventual diagnosis to the peer teachers. So in a case about abdominal pain, the mini lecture could be about the difference between Crohn's disease and ulcerative colitis. Peer teachers need to be provided with clear instructions what the mini lecture should be about. Moreover, since it is a *mini* lecture, the talk should be limited to essentials.]

Hints for peer teachers

[The mini lecture is meant to provide the students with information they can directly apply in the continuation of the case. Peer teachers should therefore make sure that the information in the mini lecture is directly applicable (i.e. explanation about pathophysiology or pros and cons of certain diagnostics). The mini lecture is by no means meant for the peer teachers to comprehensively show how much they know, but it is meant to teach the students. Peer teachers should make sure the information reaches the students.]

Background information for the consultant

[Since the consultant might not be a specialist on the subject, basic background information should be provided. The background information provided for the consultant may be more extensive than what the peer teachers are going to tell.

Consultants should also be instructed that the goal of the mini lecture is not to examine the peer teachers like in an oral examination but to let the peer teachers teach the students.]

Question 8   Try to Estimate What the Investigation Costs Are in Terms of Burden for the Patient and Cost for the Hospital

[This question is optional and meant to train students in decision-making from a different perspective than pure medical.]

Hints for peer teachers

[Peer teachers can be referred to literature.]

Background information for the consultant

[Give summarized information for the consultant.]

Stage IV: The Results of Diagnostic Tests Are Provided

Handout 3
(shown on the screen and read out loud)
   [Peer teachers distribute a handout with the findings from all diagnostic tests (text in italics). Results are given including their units and reference values. Radiological results or ECG results may be given as images as well, but peer teachers may need hints how to interpret and discuss them.
   Depending on the case, some new results of advanced diagnostic tests be provided later, if it appears to be necessary to do further investigations a later stage.]

Question 9   Interpret the Findings from the Diagnostic Tests. How Much Certainty Do They Give About the Hypotheses?

Hints for peer teachers
[Peer teachers may try to discuss specificity and sensitivity of these diagnostic tests; hints may lead them to do so. Also students may be asked to discuss if results that are slightly high/low still influence the differential diagnosis.]

Background information for the consultant
[Consultants are provided with evidence-based answers if possible.]

Question 10   Which Diagnosis Prevails Now?

Hints for peer teachers
[Peer teachers don't need many hints here.]

Background information for the consultant
[Consultants should be provided with the answer, sometimes with arguments.]

Question 11   Given this diagnosis and patient circumstances, which therapy or policy for care is now indicated? What is the prognosis if the patient is treated? What if the patient would not be treated?

Hints for peer teachers
[Peer teachers can be given hints, i.e. *think of non-pharmaceutical or pharmaceutical options/does the patient have any prehistory that makes a certain therapy more suitable/is there a difference in prognosis on the short (24 h) and long term (3 months)?*]

Background information for the consultant
[Consultants are provided with the correct answers.]

Mini Lecture by One of the Peer Teachers
[Usually only one mini lecture is given during a case as it decreases the time left for clinical reasoning. This could, however, also be a good place to insert a mini lecture

if it is about therapy options with pros and cons for each option. (Instructions how to write a mini-lecture are given after question 7.)

One of the peer teachers gives a short presentation about relevant therapy options.]

Role-Play **The information about the required or suggested therapy is conveyed to the patient. One of the students is the doctor; one of the peer teachers plays the patient. Try to explain the cause of the disease in clear language and the reason for the proposed therapy in understandable words. The other students listen and may comment afterwards.**

[A role-play is optional but can be interesting in case of a difficult or controversial investigation or therapy. A role-play should not take more than 5 min and should not focus on empathy and communication skills (which takes too long and other courses are more suitable for such competency objectives) but on the skill to summarize the medical problem in plain words. Role-plays are not frequently used in CBCR cases.]

Stage V: Information Is Provided About the Results of the Therapy Policy

Handout 4
(shown on the screen and read out loud)
[Peer teachers read out loud the therapy that has been given and the effects of it on the patient's condition over a period of time. The information in the handout is written as a story. Depending on the particular situation and the educational objective, the CBCR case may continue if the therapy is followed by a renewed presentation of the patient.]

Question 12 **One of the students from the group summarizes the whole case chronologically in a few minutes**

[This question is meant to train student to summarize cases in an efficient way, as they will often have to do this in the clinical years. It also urges students to keep alert during the whole session.

It is possible to make a distinction between an oral and written summary since an oral summary only contains a minimum of information but a written summary might also contain negative findings for this patient, which allows supervisors to know that the student has asked the patient for it. Less advanced students can use a mnemonic aid to summarize, while more advanced students should be able to give a case summary in two to three sentences.

Hint for the peer-teachers
[If necessary, students may be helped to summarize using the format.

During the office hour I saw a ... year old male/female with complaints of... As relevant prehistory I mention... Relevant medication is ....

The major problem during the history is ... During the physical examination we saw ... Additional tests showed ... (special findings or no findings). In conclusion, we saw a ... year old male/female with probably ... (work diagnosis) for which we want to start... (additional testing or policy). In the differential diagnosis we still think of...]

Scenario B

Suppose that the results of the Stage IV diagnostic test were different.
[Peer teachers now optionally present a different Stage IV handout, and the questions and the case develop in a different direction. Alternative scenarios may start at any stage II, III, or IV, but should always be compatible with the initial stage I.]

*****

It takes time to write a proper CBCR case – think of a day to a week – but great cases can be used many times and year after year. The Utrecht habit is to collect evaluation data about cases to rewrite and improve cases every year. With multiple institutions applying the CBCR method, exchange of cases is recommended. In some cases senior medical students may be asked to draft a case in the area of their interest. Experienced clinicians may edit such cases for accuracy. A high quality CBCR case should be regarded as scholarly output of a clinician educator, similar to a research paper by a clinician.

References

Dolmans, D., et al. (1997). Seven principles of effective case design for a problem-based curriculum. *Medical Teacher, 19*(3), 185–189.

Kim, S., et al. (2006). A conceptual framework for developing teaching cases: A review and synthesis of the literature across disciplines. *Medical Education, 40*(9), 867–876.

Schmidt, H. G., Rotgans, J. I., & Yew, E. H. J. (2011). The process of problem-based learning: What works and why. *Medical Education, 45*(8), 792–806.

Open Access This chapter is licensed under the terms of the Creative Commons Attribution 4.0 International License (http://creativecommons.org/licenses/by/4.0/), which permits use, sharing, adaptation, distribution and reproduction in any medium or format, as long as you give appropriate credit to the original author(s) and the source, provide a link to the Creative Commons license and indicate if changes were made.

The images or other third party material in this chapter are included in the chapter's Creative Commons license, unless indicated otherwise in a credit line to the material. If material is not included in the chapter's Creative Commons license and your intended use is not permitted by statutory regulation or exceeds the permitted use, you will need to obtain permission directly from the copyright holder.

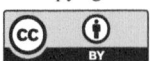

8 Writing CBCR Cases

It is possible to make a distinction between an oral and written summary since an oral summary only contains a minimum of information but a written summary might also contain negative findings for this patient, which allows supervisors to know that the student has asked the patient for it. Less advanced students can use a mnemonic aid to summarize, while more advanced students should be able to give a case summary in two to three sentences.

Hint for the peer-teachers
[If necessary, students may be helped to summarize using the format.

During the office hour I saw a ... year old male/female with complaints of... As relevant prehistory I mention... Relevant medication is ....

The major problem during the history is ... During the physical examination we saw ... Additional tests showed ... (special findings or no findings). In conclusion, we saw a ... year old male/female with probably ... (work diagnosis) for which we want to start... (additional testing or policy). In the differential diagnosis we still think of...]

Scenario B

Suppose that the results of the Stage IV diagnostic test were different.
[Peer teachers now optionally present a different Stage IV handout, and the questions and the case develop in a different direction. Alternative scenarios may start at any stage II, III, or IV, but should always be compatible with the initial stage I.]

*****

It takes time to write a proper CBCR case – think of a day to a week – but great cases can be used many times and year after year. The Utrecht habit is to collect evaluation data about cases to rewrite and improve cases every year. With multiple institutions applying the CBCR method, exchange of cases is recommended. In some cases senior medical students may be asked to draft a case in the area of their interest. Experienced clinicians may edit such cases for accuracy. A high quality CBCR case should be regarded as scholarly output of a clinician educator, similar to a research paper by a clinician.

References

Dolmans, D., et al. (1997). Seven principles of effective case design for a problem-based curriculum. *Medical Teacher, 19*(3), 185–189.

Kim, S., et al. (2006). A conceptual framework for developing teaching cases: A review and synthesis of the literature across disciplines. *Medical Education, 40*(9), 867–876.

Schmidt, H. G., Rotgans, J. I., & Yew, E. H. J. (2011). The process of problem-based learning: What works and why. *Medical Education, 45*(8), 792–806.

Open Access This chapter is licensed under the terms of the Creative Commons Attribution 4.0 International License (http://creativecommons.org/licenses/by/4.0/), which permits use, sharing, adaptation, distribution and reproduction in any medium or format, as long as you give appropriate credit to the original author(s) and the source, provide a link to the Creative Commons license and indicate if changes were made.

The images or other third party material in this chapter are included in the chapter's Creative Commons license, unless indicated otherwise in a credit line to the material. If material is not included in the chapter's Creative Commons license and your intended use is not permitted by statutory regulation or exceeds the permitted use, you will need to obtain permission directly from the copyright holder.

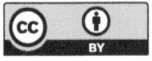

Chapter 9
Curriculum, Course, and Faculty Development for Case-Based Clinical Reasoning

Olle ten Cate and Gaiane Simonia

The current chapter gives a brief overview of the conditions for developing a modern curriculum for medical education to include CBCR and about faculty development for CBCR teachers. The introduction of CBCR is only one element of a full curriculum; yet, just as a complete curriculum, it requires careful planning.

A Brief Introduction to Curriculum Development

"Curriculum," sometimes simply defined as "a planned educational experience" (Thomas et al. 2016), has evolved as a concept to be applied to several levels of education: a macrolevel (requirements defined by a government for an accredited or subsidized course), a meso-level (a plan for a school with university rules and methods of teaching and assessment), and a microlevel (an instrument to guide a classroom teacher in determining content and methods to be used in individual lessons). While this is informative, it still is very general. Janet Grant proposed that a curriculum is "a statement of the intended aims and objectives, content, experiences, outcomes and processes of an educational program, including a description of the training structure and of the expected methods of learning, teaching, feedback and supervision" (Grant 2010). To be even more practical, Mulder and ten Cate, based on extensive experience with curriculum development, constructed a ten-element

---

O. ten Cate (✉)
Center for Research and Development of Education, University Medical Center Utrecht, Utrecht, The Netherlands
e-mail: T.J.tenCate@umcutrecht.nl

G. Simonia
Tbilisi State Medical University, Tbilisi, Georgia
e-mail: gsimonia@gmail.com

definition that can guide educators embarking on major curriculum innovation projects (Mulder and ten Cate 2006). A full curriculum description, in this approach, includes a mission statement, objectives, a description of intended learners, an educational philosophy, a general curriculum framework, descriptions of individual units or courses, methods of assessment with rules on student progress and examinations, an organizational and management structure, clear conditions for teaching personnel, finances and facilities, and a quality assurance structure. All of these deserve a much wider elaboration, but for the purpose of this book, we will confine the description to Table 9.1.

These elements comply with international standards for medical curricula (Lindgren 2012). However, it should be realized that a curriculum is a living thing that is only effective in the way it is delivered by teachers and received by students. Authors have distinguished the *planned* curriculum (as exemplified above), the *delivered* curriculum (as understood and carried out by teachers), the *experienced* curriculum (as perceived by students), and even a *hidden* curriculum (not reflected in formal rules and intentions but conveyed implicitly by the unwritten rules and observed behaviors) (Prideaux 2003; Hafferty and Franks 1994). We cannot and should not avoid differences between these "curricula" but must be aware of them and cautious that pathways students follow, even if not designed by curriculum developers, are effective in their learning toward common goals of medical education. There are many "pathways to Rome," and, around the world, there are many routes to the medical degree (Wijnen-Meijer et al. 2013). There is not one "best" curriculum, and the success of a curriculum is very dependent on the students who follow it and the local and national context. Students' motivation to become a doctor can make them just do anything that seems appropriate to get the degree, no matter what curriculum or even in which country or jurisdiction. This individual intrinsic motivation should be valued and stimulated, even with their deviations from a planned path, as long as student creativity is constructive for their own career development (ten Cate et al. 2011).

The Process of Curriculum Development

The curriculum development process for medical education is originally well described by Kern and colleagues from Johns Hopkins University School of Medicine, now revised by Thomas et al (2016). In elaborate and widely used guidelines, the authors recommend to committees embarking on a curriculum development process, to follow "Kern six steps" (slightly adapted):

1. *Problem identification and general needs assessment*: Why is change necessary? What health problems in society have priority in a new curriculum?
2. *Needs assessment of targeted learners*: Curricula will work best if students feel motivated to spend effort in learning, so identify them and query them.

9 Curriculum, Course, and Faculty Development for Case-Based Clinical Reasoning

Table 9.1 Ten elements that constitute a curriculum description

	Element	Description
1	Mission statement	This is a carefully stated, well-considered rationale, no longer than one paragraph that summarizes the overall intention of the curriculum.
2	Objectives	An overview is provided of the learning goals of the curriculum, preferably meeting the needs of society on a national level, thus reflecting what graduates must have mastered. Elaborate objective frameworks, such as derived from Bloom can be found on the Internet (Bloom et al. 1956).
3	Intended learners and admission policy	The type of students and their backgrounds that the school desires to attract, including criteria for selection and admission, are described.
4	Educational philosophy	This paragraph shows how the curriculum committee grounds decisions of the practical implementation and may include aspects of educational theory, integration, problem-based approach, and views on clinical teaching.
5	Curriculum framework	Visualization of the curriculum is important to communicate with all faculty and students involved in planning and delivering the curriculum. A chart showing all individual curriculum units, arranged by weeks of the year (vertically) and program years (horizontally) and by color to signify unit types is often used.
6	Individual units	Each unit, sometimes called course or module, must be described as a micro curriculum in itself with objectives and methods of teaching and assessment.
7	Methods of assessment and rules on progress and exams	Assessment approaches can be derived from Miller's pyramid (Miller 1990) and should include written (or electronic) tests, standardized skills assessment, and methods of assessment in the clinical environment. Important are rules for progression of learners, as this is what concerns many students most when they follow a curriculum; these rules should be carefully designed to stimulate learning in the direction of the real goals of education.
8	Governance, coordination, and administration	A powerful curriculum governance structure must be in place to guarantee collaboration of departments, integration where necessary, and quality control. Tasks for program and course directors should be specified. Student and examination data must be efficiently collected and stored. A central medical education unit is highly recommended.
9	Funding and facilities	Conditional for high-quality education is sufficient funding for teaching time and support, and physical facilities, such as suitable classrooms, internet and library access, and a skills lab.
10	Quality assurance and faculty development	Every curriculum must continuously be monitored for its quality and modified if needed. *Plan-do-check-act* is a well-known cycle that can establish the foundation for a curriculum quality assurance procedure. Teachers should be trained and qualified to teach, particularly when the education is not identical to their own education. Understanding the learning process of students is crucial for effective student-centered education (ten Cate et al. 2004). Teachers in medical schools must be provided time to teach and rewarded for high-quality teaching.

3. *Goals and objectives*: Specific and measurable learner objectives, behaviorally formulated, will help to monitor progress of students.
4. *Educational strategies*: Objectives should lead to the choice of suitable methods of teaching to attain these objectives.
5. *Implementation*: Starting a new curriculum involves identifying resources; obtaining support, administrative structures, and communication strategy; anticipating barriers to change, and piloting before full implementation.
6. *Evaluation and feedback*: This includes the identification of users, resources, and issues that circulate, to design procedures and questions, choose or construct measurement instruments, collect and analyze data, and efficiently report results, feeding into a new cycle of quality assurance.

This summary combines a process that may take years to prepare and execute, but all steps are important. Two decades ago Gale and Grant compiled an AMEE Guide that is still extremely helpful in change management for medical curricula (Gale and Grant 1997).

Course Development for CBCR

Introducing just CBCR on top of a medical curriculum that already exists is possible and does not require a major organizational change in infrastructure and a long timeline to fundamentally reform a full undergraduate program. In fact, the introduction of a CBCR course following the format presented in this book can be relatively simple. However, a case-based clinical reasoning course as described in earlier chapters exemplifies many of the characteristic of what has been called a "modern" medical curriculum, since an acronym for that (SPICES) was introduced in the 1980s (Harden et al. 1984): Student centered (particularly through the peer teaching approach), Problem based (clinical problems are the focus), Integrated (its differential diagnostic approach crosses the boundaries of clinical specialties, and applied basic science can be incorporated), Community based (depending on the cases used, this can be a focus), elective (the course is usually mandatory but can be elective), and Systematic (CBCR is an example of a very systematic approach to clinical education). Introducing CBCR in an existing traditional curriculum, as has been done in several Eastern-European countries, can be a first step to a school acquainted with modern approaches to medical education.

In Table 9.2 steps for course development are suggested, with reference to both Kern's six-step approach and the definition of a curriculum given earlier. As CBCR is only a course, the development is simplified.

The implementation of a new CBCR course should be planned well ahead. Particularly the writing of high-quality cases can take much more time than one would initially think or hope. Some clinicians are excellent, naturally born case writers; others need a lot of assistance and editing support. Given the fact that many will do this in spare hours, the planning ahead of a new CBCR course should take at least one full year before the real start.

Table 9.2 Elements of CBCR course development and implementation

1	*Educational needs assessment*
	The school must feel the need to introduce CBCR, so some effort to assess this need is helpful to secure support and a general agreement before starting the course development. This need could be (a) the wish of clinical teachers to see students better prepared when they must take up patient care responsibilities. Clinical reasoning is at the core of health care, and students must be well trained to think like a doctor; (b) just the wish to experiment with curriculum modernization without an early disruption of the full existing curriculum. Introducing CBCR can very well be this first step before a more systematic creation of an integrated curriculum; or (c) a wish from students or science faculty to integrate basic science education more with clinical thinking.
	The needs assessment can be simply carried out by structured interviews or a questionnaire among carefully selected stakeholders (clinicians, basic scientists, students). A clear, concise report may ease the way to a decision by the right body (committee, dean, board) to proceed with the course development.
2	*Content needs assessment and objectives*
	A content needs assessment gives an answer to the question: *which pathology has the priority to be translated in CBCR cases to be discussed and learned and, more detailed, in which curriculum year?* Basically CBCR can be introduced in the first curriculum year in a very integrated curriculum, but, as prior knowledge is applied in case discussions, students must have relevant prior knowledge. We recommend starting CBCR from the second year or later with cases that can increase in complexity. CBCR is meant as preparation for clinical rotations. Depending on the curriculum, CBCR can extend over the 2nd and 3rd and even 4th and sometimes even 5th year. The nature of a preclinical course will then be adapted, but the format can remain the same.
	Sources of information can be health statistics of the population of the country or of hospitals and practices. Cases for CBCR should reflect a broad range of relevant common medical conditions that have educational value.
3	*Intended learners*
	A decision should be made which students should follow this course and, in addition, how long and when the course is to be scheduled. In most cases it will be a mandatory course for all students, but in an initial pilot phase, it can be offered as an elective course.
4	*General course framework*
	This plan – for a full curriculum, this would be called a blueprint – can be summarized on two pages and should include the general objectives, case titles, number and duration of sessions, the clinical disciplines involved and number of cases per discipline, the origin of the cases (written by own faculty or derived from other sources, such as this book), size and number of student groups, rough scheduling (e.g., one session per 2 weeks at a suitable time), physical requirements (number of small-group class rooms needed), number of teachers (consultants) needed, and from which disciplines.
5	*Method of assessment and examination rules*
	This section of the plan should stipulate how many credits the course offers (in European credits, 5 sessions could be 1 EC, provided that these would include 1 peer teacher assignment), how satisfactory participation is awarded, and how acquired knowledge and skills are tested. Based on our experience, we recommend that 10–15 % of the final score is determined by active participation and 85–90 % on a written (or electronic) test.

(continued)

Table 9.2 (continued)

6	Coordination and teachers
	The coordination of the course should reside with a course director or course coordinator, preferably formally appointed by the dean or by a curriculum director. Consultants (teachers) from different clinical departments should be involved. It is a benefit if case writers also act as consultants, as this enables them to see how their case works out in practice and how the case can be improved if necessary. Consultants should be attached to a group for the full course, which means that they will not just guide the group within their own specialty. Given the consultant text version available and their general medical knowledge, preparation for a session is very feasible for nonexpert doctors. UMC Utrecht even has very favorable experience with senior medical students just before graduation acting as CBCR consultants (Zijdenbos et al. 2010). It is advised that the course director has a meeting at least once a year with all consultants.
7	Funding
	Funding of courses is organized very differently across schools, but as with any program, teachers should be available for both the course hours and its development and preparation. As a rule of thumb: writing a case should be calculated as 1 full week of work (40 h), updating the case about 6 h per year. A full course of 10 CBCR sessions should be awarded as 40 h per consultant (per session 2 contact hours and 2 preparation hours, which include correspondence and meetings). Preparing, administering, and analyzing exams can be estimated about an hour per student on average. Coordination by the course director may be calculated as 4–6 h per group per year. A quick calculation of the required funding per year for a full 10-session course for 300 students working in groups of 12 would amount to 400 h once and 1,600 h annually. Breakdown:
	- Development of cases: 400 h (only once)
	- Annual case updates: 60 h
	- Annual coordination: 140 h
	- Annual consultant effort: 1,000 h
	- Annual effort preparing, administering, processing exams: 300 h
	- Annual administration (student data, materials, evaluation): 100 h
	In addition, regular course administration printed materials and facilities require a limited budget. The consultant effort clearly requires the biggest funding, comparable with PBL funding. As said, however, junior doctors can be excellent consultants, if provided with high-quality cases and proper guidance, which would significantly lower costs.
8	Program evaluation
	A system of continuous course improvement should be devised. This should include the collection of information directly after sessions about case quality (what can be improved?), from both consultants and students, and also student information about teacher quality (how can faculty improve their teaching skills?) and about facilities (rooms, communication, organization). A curriculum program director can have an annual interview with the CBCR course director based on evaluation data and agree upon actions for next year.

The Aim of Faculty Development

Most faculty members of medical schools and medical universities have been trained to be adequate clinicians or scientists or both. Only a minority, although growing, has been trained to be a teacher, and it is odd to realize that as education gets more sophisticated – from grade school to university – fewer requirements apply for teaching skills.

Table 9.3 UMC Utrecht's model of teaching certificates for faculty

	Certificate or diploma	Target group
1	Student teaching certificate	Optional for senior medical students choosing an elective teaching rotation (ten Cate 2007)
2	Teaching certificate	Required for all faculty members
3	Advanced teaching certificate	Required for senior faculty in leadership roles
4	Postgraduate scholarly educator certificate	Optional for senior medical educators who aspire a career in scholarship of education
5	PhD diploma in health professions education research	For those educators aspiring to become researchers of education in the health professions

If teaching would remain identical over the years, teachers could learn the tricks of the trade from their colleagues and remember how they themselves received education. But in a rapidly changing world, education has become quite different by the time students are faculty members themselves and must start teaching students.

Medical educators around the world begin to agree that faculty must be trained before they should be allowed to teach, just as students cannot treat patients if not properly trained. In practice this is too strict a rule, but universities have started requiring new faculty to obtain a basic teaching certificate and an advanced certification for teachers in leadership positions. Table 9.3 shows the model that exists at the University Medical Center Utrecht as an example.

An elaborate framework of teaching competencies for medical educators is provided by Molenaar et al. (2009) and establishes an excellent grounding for faculty development. It distinguishes teaching domains (development, organization, execution, coaching, assessment, and program evaluation) and levels of responsibility (leadership, coordination, and actual teaching – macro-meso-micro), resulting in many detailed teaching competencies that deserve attention in trainings.

Faculty Development for CBCR

Faculty development just for a CBCR course is limited but necessary, and we recommend that it exists of the four components mentioned in Table 9.4.

The following section describes a case study of the introduction of CBCR in a Post-Soviet country. This curriculum and faculty development initiative was part of the EU-Tempus project Modernizing Undergraduate Medical Education in the Eastern Neighboring Area (MUMEENA) of the EU, carried out in the years 2011–2014.

Table 9.4 Components of faculty development for CBCR

1	*Written instructions*
	Written instructions about the background and practicalities of cases-based clinical reasoning education. This book can serve as the resource for this.
2	*Training of case writers*
	One strategy that has been used is to ask writers to make a first draft of a case based on the detailed guidelines in this book, present these drafts before a group of colleague case writers during a workshop, and ask for comments. Group discussions about the level of detail, related to the target group of students, are often very helpful. The session could be one afternoon (3–4 h with a 30 min break), and one case discussion could be 10 mins of presentation, followed by 20 mins of guided discussion in a group of six case writers. Next, multiple writers could be formed to mutually review and edit each other's cases over the course of some weeks to come. One coordinator, preferably a future course director, could be involved in the final editing of the case for consistency across cases.
3	*Training of consultants*
	Several instructional modes have been used. One is the creation and use of a film that shows the process of CBCR from the student perspective. That is quite an investment if done properly, but the result can be very instructive for new faculty members preparing to act as consultants. Another option is to observe a group while actually delivering a CBCR session. What is needed is a room that provides accommodation not only for the group and its consultant but also for an outer ring of observing faculty. It is helpful to have an experienced educator facilitate this process and apply a *time-in time-out* procedure. This means that the group proceeds with a regular CBCR session until the facilitator calls for a time-out, to allow for comments, questions, and answers from the outer ring audience, after which the group continues. Finally, didactic techniques to deal with group dynamic processes may be a topic for the training for all types of small-group teaching, including CBCR. See Fig. 9.1 for an example.
4	*Training of students*
	While strictly not faculty development, the instruction of students is important too. Even students have a teaching role, as they all must act as a peer teacher for multiple sessions. Specifically students who have no experience with open group discussions and those who are afraid to provide wrong answers in classroom sessions must develop a new mindset. Education of students is to help to correct mistakes, and only by asking about things students do *not* know, i.e., disclosing their ignorance, they can be corrected. CBCR is very much student centered and student driven, and this role may be very new for students. Before a first CBCR session and during a first session, there should be much space to discuss the procedural aspects of CBCR.

Case Study: Introducing CBCR at Tbilisi State Medical University, Georgia

As part of a project to modernize medical education in Eastern Europe, in 2011 a 3-year EU-funded project included the introduction of CBCR at six universities in three countries, one of which was Georgia. The following steps were taken:

1. *Introduction of the CBCR rationale and concepts*

    In January 2012, a workshop conducted by educators from UMC Utrecht, The Netherlands, was held at Tbilisi State Medical University (TSMU) to have faculty learn for the first time about this method and its significance for curriculum innovation. Previous evaluations of existing teaching methods had shown that graduates experience serious difficulties in clinical decision-making during residency. The workshop resulted in a proposal to select ten common medical

9 Curriculum, Course, and Faculty Development for Case-Based Clinical Reasoning 117

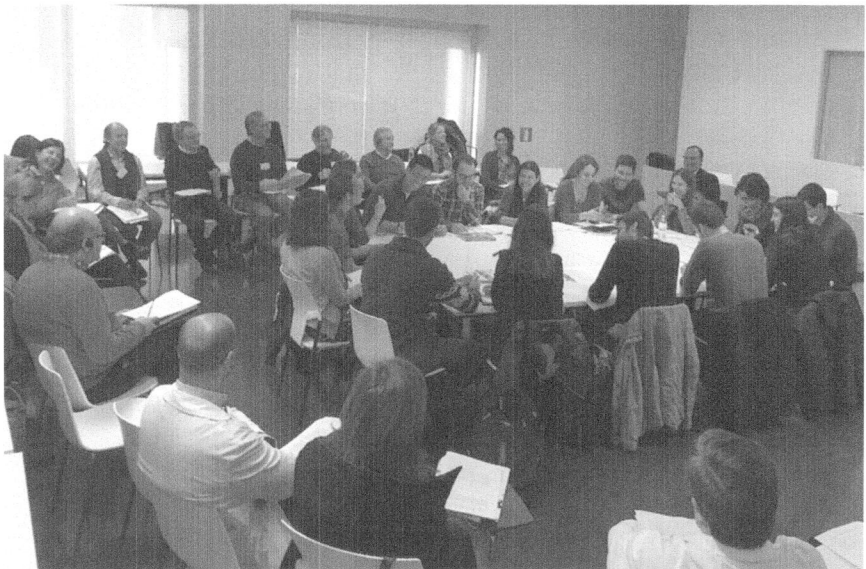

Fig. 9.1 A faculty development session at the University of Granada School of Medicine (2017) showing the demonstration of a CBCR session conducted by medical students, while faculty members are observing

conditions for elaboration in CBCR cases (swollen legs, cough, breathlessness, abdominal pain, loss of consciousness, arthralgia, urine incontinence, jaundice, tiredness, chest pain). It was also decided to introduce an extracurricular pilot CBCR course for third year students – at the so-called "preclinical" stage.

2. *Training in case writing and demonstration of CBCR*

    In March 2012, 10 active and enthusiastic faculty members, all of them clinicians and considered as prospective CBCR teachers (consultants), were trained during 1 week in CBCR methodology at the University Medical Center Utrecht, The Netherlands. The training focused on case writing and a demonstration of CBCR in practice by Utrecht medical students was given.

3. *Pilot introduction of CBCR and evaluation*

    Preceded by 5 months piloting of 10 CBCR sessions in and following a decision of the TSMU Academic Council, CBCR was included in 2012–2013 for 10 groups (135 students) in the third year of the undergraduate medical curriculum for 2 ECTS credits. The duration of each session, delivered once a week, was 3 h. By the end of each session, questionnaires were provided to all CBCR consultants and students. This showed that 96 % of all consultants valued CBCR as a useful course for learning clinical thinking and helpful to improve students' ability to resolve clinical problems. About 84 % of the students rated the CBCR course as an excellent teaching tool, teaching them the approach and attitude toward patient problems and the methodology of differential diagnosis, and in addition improved their communication and leadership skills.

4. *Formal decision to introduce CBCR*

    Based on this positive feedback, the TSMU Academic Council decided to consider CBCR as a compulsory course for all third year TSMU students from the 2013–2014 academic year, i.e., for 500 Georgian and 250 international third year students.

5. *Spread in other universities*

    Following the successful implementation of CBCR at TSMU, the course was also introduced in partner medical schools in Azerbaijan and Ukraine, likewise supported by workshops in Kiev and Baku.

6. *Lessons learned*

    The introduction of CBCR took 2 years of preparation, negotiation, and faculty development but was clearly successful. With respect to the teaching method, feedback from students revealed, next to general satisfaction, the following points for improvement or attention:

- During CBCR sessions the mere presence of senior clinician consultants can suppress student activity, in particular, communication initiative of peer teachers, clearly a further issue for teacher training.
- Not rarely, consultants tried to unduly interfere with case discussions in the group – another issue for training.
- There were sessions when students were less active, while peer teachers tried to recall previously memorized texts from their written materials – student instruction must stress their roles.
- Due to a yet limited number of CBCR case scenarios, it was not always possible to avoid disclosure of correct answers (i.e., diagnoses) to other students' groups if their session was scheduled at different times; it reveals the anxiety students feel to not know the "right" answer. Students must learn to understand that the reasoning process is just as important as the right answer.
- Several students have suggested to become involved in the CBCR case writing process themselves.

In sum, faculty development is important, but, as this example shows, it can be very successful.

References

Bloom, B., et al. (1956). *Taxonomy of educational objectives: The classification of educational goals; handbook I: Cognitive domain.* New York: Longmans, Green.

Gale, R., & Grant, J. (1997). AMEE medical education guide no. 10: Managing change in a medical context: Guidelines for action. *Medical Teacher, 19*(4), 239–249.

Grant, J. (2010). Principles of curriculum design. In *Understanding medical education* (pp. 1–15). Chichester: Wiley-Blackwell.

Hafferty, F., & Franks, R. (1994). The hidden curriculum, ethics teaching, and the structure of medical education. *Academic Medicine, 69*(11), 861–171.

Harden, R. M., Sowden, S., & Dunn, W. (1984). Educational strategies in curriculum development: The SPICES model. *Medical Education, 18*, 284–297.

Lindgren S. (2012). *Basic medical education WFME global standards for quality improvement – the 2012 revision*. Copenhagen. Available at: http://www.wfme.org/standards/bme

Miller, G. E. (1990). The assessment of clinical skills/competence/performance. *Academic Medicine, 87*(7), S63–S67.

Molenaar, W., et al. (2009). A framework of teaching competencies across the medical education continuum. *Medical Teacher, 31*, 390–396.

Mulder, H., & ten Cate, O. (2006). *Curricular innovation as a project. (Curriculuminnovatie als project) [Dutch]*. Groningen: Wolters-Noordhoff.

Prideaux, D. (2003). Curriculum design. *British Medical Journal, 326*(February), 268–270.

ten Cate, O. (2007). A teaching rotation and a student teaching qualification for senior medical students. *Medical Teacher, 29*(6), 566–571.

ten Cate, O., et al. (2004). Orienting teaching toward the learning process. *Academic Medicine: Journal of the Association of American Medical Colleges, 79*(3), 219–228.

ten Cate, O., Kusurkar, R. A., & Williams, G. C. (2011). How self-determination theory can assist our understanding of the teaching and learning processes in medical education. AMEE guide no. 59. *Medical Teacher, 33*(12), 961–973.

Thomas, P., et al. (2016). *Curriculum development for medical education* (3rd ed.). Baltimore: The Johns Hopkins University Press.

Wijnen-Meijer, M., et al. (2013). Stages and transitions in medical education around the world: Clarifying structures and terminology. *Medical Teacher, 35*(4), 301–307.

Zijdenbos, I. L., et al. (2010). A student-led course in clinical reasoning in the core curriculum. *International Journal of Medical Education, 1*, 42–46.

Open Access This chapter is licensed under the terms of the Creative Commons Attribution 4.0 International License (http://creativecommons.org/licenses/by/4.0/), which permits use, sharing, adaptation, distribution and reproduction in any medium or format, as long as you give appropriate credit to the original author(s) and the source, provide a link to the Creative Commons license and indicate if changes were made.

The images or other third party material in this chapter are included in the chapter's Creative Commons license, unless indicated otherwise in a credit line to the material. If material is not included in the chapter's Creative Commons license and your intended use is not permitted by statutory regulation or exceeds the permitted use, you will need to obtain permission directly from the copyright holder.

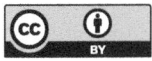

Chapter 10
A Model Study Guide for Case-Based Clinical Reasoning

Maria van Loon, Sjoukje van den Broek, and Olle ten Cate

Student Instructions and Background Materials for the CBCR Group Meetings

Authors: [name, role, affiliation, office, telephone for contact]
Year: [year of validity of the guide]

Table of Contents
- Justification
- Coordination
- Credit points

1. Introduction
2. The Objectives of the CBCR Course
3. What Is Clinical Reasoning and Decision-Making?
4. The CBCR Sessions
5. Assessment
    5.1 CBCR Session Participation Points
    5.2 The CBCR Test
    5.3 Rules for Test Participation and Passing
    5.4 Rules for the Exam Retake
    5.5 Rules for Repeaters

Justification
[Names of case writers and developers of the course.]

Coordinating team
[Names and affiliations of course director and team members; contact information of the coordination team.]

Credit Points
Having successfully completed the CBCR course in Year [...] provides [...] credits.

Introduction

[Gives a short general introduction on the CBCR course.]

Case-based clinical reasoning, a series of meetings on clinical decision-making, constitutes an important part of the curriculum. This education not only serves as a training in the methods of clinical decision-making but also provides an opportunity to apply previously acquired knowledge to clinical problems.

Students will learn clinical reasoning by using written clinical situations. In CBCR the complaint of the patient is the key starting point for reasoning. From this complaint, a case is worked through toward a diagnosis and sometimes proceeds to a management plan in a structured way. CBCR basically asks you to think in a way that is used later in clinical practice. The systematic unraveling of a clinical problem is essential in the practice of the profession of a doctor. In addition, working in groups does not only encourage the learning process but also stimulates to argue the diagnostic process step by step.

Between the CBCR classes there is time reserved for independent study. Preparatory self-directed learning improves the efficiency of the group meetings significantly and also distributes your study load more evenly.

The Objectives of the CBCR Course

[Describes the learning goals/objectives of the course.]

CBCR focuses on learning to solve clinical problems. By doing this, knowledge from pathophysiology, epidemiology, and clinical decision-making is integrated.

The student who has successfully completed the CBCR course is able to reason clinically and systematically on patient problems as presented in situations similar to the CBCR cases discussed. This includes:

– Evaluation of collected data and making clear how they relate to a complaint/medical problem

- Using of biomedical, epidemiological, and clinical knowledge in patient problems
- Making a focused differential diagnosis and evaluating all relevant hypotheses
- Giving a general direction which therapy and/or guidance is suitable

In addition, the student has acquired the skill to deal with new patient problems as presented at the doctor's office aligned with CBCR cases in the course.

Next, there is a focus on developing leadership skills. After successfully completing the CBCR course, the student is able to lead a meeting on clinical reasoning.

What Is Clinical Reasoning and Decision-Making?

[As students are mostly not really aware what clinical reasoning and clinical decision-making is, an explanation is necessary, illustrated by an example.]

Without giving a conclusive definition of clinical decision-making, it can be said that this form of education is about the rational considerations that underpin every step in the clinical encounter that starts at the moment when a patient presents at the doctor's office, until the moment that an end is reached in this contact.

The nature of this process is usually that of solving a medical question or problem. The considerations that guide that process are an essential part of the group discussions. The quality of the arguments, considerations, and decisions made is just as important as the solutions to be found. Many arguments include both pathophysiological and non-pathophysiological arguments. Pathophysiological arguments concern the construction and functioning of the body up to a molecular level and the disturbance of them. Non-pathophysiological arguments usually relate to epidemiological, but sometimes to ethical or social considerations. Eliminating a pathophysiological argued statement because a particular phenomenon in a certain group of people rarely occurs is an epidemiological founded argument. Also the decision not to carry out a specific diagnostic test because the costs and burden on the patient are in no proportion to the information that the doctor will receive is a non-pathophysiological argument. Clinical decision-making is schematically displayed below (Boxes 10.1 and 10.2):

The CBCR Sessions

[This is a practical section and describes how the sessions take place and what is expected of the students].

During the CBCR sessions you will work through written clinical cases in a group of students. Every session, three students take the role of peer teacher and lead the session. A consultant is present to act as supervisor.

> **Box 10.1 A Roadmap to Clinical Decision-Making**
> 1. Identify what the question(s) is/(are) of the patient. As long as the patient's request for help is not clarified, you will need to ask further questions, until it is completely clear what questions, wishes, and expectations the patient has.
> 2. After the request for help is clarified, formulate possible diagnoses before you start with history taking.
> 3. Estimate the order of likelihood of hypotheses within the differential diagnosis.
> 4. Argue every diagnosis with pathophysiological and non-pathophysiological arguments.
> 5. Schematically confirm or reject all possible diagnoses.
>   (a) What next history question should you ask? What does an answer tell you?
>   (b) What next part of the physical examination would you perform? Why?
>   (c) What diagnostic tests would you now like to order?
>
> Argue every question and every diagnostic test. If you want to collect multiple data, make a priority list of what needs to be asked/done first.
>
> 6. Evaluate the data collected through history and additional research.
> 7. Repeat 3–6 until you have a most likely diagnosis and you cannot gain more certainty about the diagnosis. Then proceed to prognosis and therapy.

Introduction Session

In an introduction session, the students and their consultant get acquainted with each other. The consultant explains the purposes of CBCR course and gives the instructions for the sessions. Rules and regulations are set. The first three peer teachers are chosen, and they receive the peer teacher version of the first case.

Preparation and Self-Study

A distinction is made between the preparation of the students and the peer teachers. The peer teachers (three students rotating in the group) prepare the case thoroughly in advance so that they are able to lead the meeting. All other students prepare the meeting at home with the student version of the case. This preparation is necessary to ascertain a high-level discussion. All cases can be prepared using the prescribed literature given in the cases.

Box 10.2 Example Case Using the Roadmap for Clinical Decision-Making

A 35-year-old woman visits the family doctor because she is so tired lately during exercise. She also reports that she loses a lot of blood during her menstruation. You check her hemoglobin level; this is 6.2 mmol/L.

- ad 1   The request for help might be: "What is the cause of my fatigue?"
- ad 2   The first assumption in this case is obvious: Is the heavy menstruation the cause of the anemia and, therefore, the fatigue with exertion? What possible causes of anemia are there?

1. Disorder in the production
2. Loss of blood
3. Hemolytic anemia

- ad 3/4   An iron-deficiency anemia based on a heavy menstruation is most likely based on the following arguments:

1. Epidemiological argument: Iron-deficiency anemia is by far the most common.
2. Pathophysiological argument: A heavy menstruation can indeed lead to anemia.

- ad 5a   Deepening the history with special history questions is not very burdensome. Yet efficiency is desired. So it is wise to ask first for her menstruation cycle. Asking for blood with defecation (in case of suspicion on a bowel tumor) comes later in the hierarchy. Of course, you should also ask about other causes of fatigue with exertion, for example, complaints matching asthma – you know that anemia does not always give complaints of fatigue.
- ad 5b   There is also a hierarchy in the physical examination. A gynecological examination gives us probably more information than a rectal examination (a fibroid in the uterus is sometimes felt better than a tumor in the rectum).
- ad 5c   Many different diagnostic tests can be done to determine the cause of the anemia, such as MCV, hematocrit, and ferritin. However, it is important for each test to be aware of the (cost) effectiveness. MCV and hematocrit are cheap, not very stressful, and deliver a significant diagnostic result. However, a colonoscopy is expensive and stressful, and the chance that this patient has a carcinoma is small.

CBCR Sessions

Each session takes 2 h,[1] and during these sessions, patient cases will be discussed, increasing in difficulty over the course.

The aim of each session is to elaborate a clinical problem. At first a hypothesis or differential diagnosis is formulated after a patient problem has been introduced. This is elaborated by asking relevant questions on the problem and to test the first hypotheses. Too much or unfocused questioning means that the process is not well finished. The process of formulating and testing hypotheses is repeated one or more times after additional information is provided by means of "handouts" that include information of the history, the physical examination, imaging tests, and/or specified laboratory research. Before the sessions, only the peer teachers have handout information, which they will distribute during the class. Afterward, the handouts will be available for all students.

Tasks of Peer Teachers

Peer teacher roles for the first and subsequent sessions are assigned at the introduction session. By turn, at each session three students perform the role of peer teacher; every student fulfills this role at least twice[2] during the course. Peer teachers lead CBCR meetings. They have prepared the case using the peer teacher version of the case, which they have received from the consultant at the end of the previous session. This version of the case provides additional hints for the peer teachers. As a result, they are able to work through the complete case before the session, lead the discussion in the meeting, give comments on the arguments of other group members, and provide well-funded answers. During the session one of the peer teachers gives a mini-lecture to provide the students with additional information about a certain diagnosis, test, or therapy. The instructions for this are given in the peer teacher's version.

The overall course of the meeting is as follows:

- *Introduction*: Introduction of the patient and formulation of the patient problem.
- *Answering*: Answering of the first questions by every student or in little groups (2–3 students).
- *Inventory of the answers*: Especially the arguments are important.

---

[1] Duration of the sessions depends on local schedules. We advise a minimum duration of 1.45 and a maximum of 2.30 h.

[2] Depending on the number of sessions and number of students per group. This is an example of the situation at the University Medical Center Utrecht.

- *Reflection on the responses*: Reflection on the responses by the peer teachers and explanation of what they think that the proper responses are (a mini-lecture can be useful).
- *Brief summary*: At the end of the case, one of the students gives a brief summary of the patient and his/her complaint.
- *Evaluation*: The student participation is evaluated and assessed by the consultant, material for the next meeting is distributed, and the case or the meeting is discussed and evaluated.

The value of CBCR consists of the ability of students to formulate new hypotheses based on new information received. Therefore, it is very important that the students do not know in advance how the case will proceed and do not know answers on the history or diagnostics. As peer teachers you are kindly but firmly requested not to give any information concerning the case to students who haven't had this meeting yet.

Tips

Peer teachers are expected to be able to argue through all steps in the clinical decision-making of this particular case. The following tips are provided to make the peer teacher role feasible:

- Make sure that the students have answered the questions the best they can. Only then provide them with comments and additions.
- Avoid the group to become passive. Involve every student in the discussion. Even the students who haven't prepared properly can try to answer questions.
- Bring literature to the sessions. Any unforeseen questions can be answered, and a solution can be found during the session. The consultant should not be the primary source of information, but can be asked for feedback in case the group cannot continue.
- The peer teachers determine the course of the meeting. The role of the consultant can be limited if the peer teachers are well prepared.
- The peer teachers can use a whiteboard, flip over, or PowerPoint to make tables or to use it for their mini-lecture.
- Peer teachers play an important role in the evaluation of the cases. Any comments they have should be handed to the consultant.
- CBCR trains peer teachers in leadership skills. Three roles can be distinguished.

(a) The *chairperson*
    (i) Takes the lead
    (ii) Divides turns to get everyone involved (in addition actively involve silent students, e.g., let the neighbor of an answering student argue the answer given)
    (iii) Ensures time management

(b) The *summarizer*

    (i) Identifies key issues after the discussion
    (ii) Provides a conclusion at the end of a question
    (iii) Writes down keywords on the board and fills in the table

(c) The *content expert*

    (i) Is critical; is not easily satisfied with the answers given by the students
    (ii) Asks thoroughly: what does a student mean with an answer?
    (iii) Seeks answers to questions that remain unresolved on the spot, to be able to answer them before the end of the meeting.

It is important that the tasks are alternated during the meeting, since the consultant will assess peer teachers on their overall performance.

The Mini-Lecture

Mini-lectures are meant to provide students with background information to proceed with the case. The provided information must be directly applicable (i.e., explanation about diagnostic tests) or create a better understanding of a topic (i.e., explanation about pathophysiology). Tips for a good mini-lecture:

- Keep it simple in form and content
    - Form:

        Use as little text as possible on the slides
        Use images
        Use a clear structure

    - Content:

        Make sure you have an evident message and conclusion
        Be cautious with details

- Maintain contact with the group
    - Check if your message comes trough
    - Ask questions
    - Mind your voice and presentation
    - Be aware of the level of preparation of the students

N.B. The mini-lecture is not meant as a recitation for the peer teachers or merely an exposure of their content knowledge, but is meant to teach the students. Mini-lectures should not take more than about 5 min.

PowerPoint and Whiteboard

Experience has shown that the use of PowerPoint during the CBCR session can undermine the clinical thinking process. Therefore, its use should be limited to showing handout texts and to support a mini-lecture. It is advised to use the blackboard or whiteboard as much as possible in the interactive discussions on hypotheses and disease symptoms. Building a clear table (with diagnostic hypotheses and diagnostic findings on the two axes) helps with structuring a reflective thinking process.

Tasks of Regular Students

All students are expected to be prepared and show active participation in the meetings.

Tasks of the Consultant

The main task of the consultant is to encourage the students to have a meaningful discussion about the clinical problem. He or she acts as a supervisor. As for the provision of content knowledge, the teacher is a true consultant, reacting to student requests for information if needed. In addition, the consultant's task is to assess the active participation of all students. The consultant gives feedback, especially to the peer teachers.

At the end of the session, as an administrative task, the consultant hands out the peer teacher versions to the peer teachers for the next session.

Assessment

[Gives information on assessment of group meeting and final assessment of the course and general rules on missing sessions]

The course requirements include both active participation at sessions as students and as peer teachers and passing the CBCR test. Participation makes up 12 % and the test score 88 % of the final mark.[3]

---

[3] This is an example of the University Medical Center Utrecht, where participation during sessions makes 12 % and the test score 88 % of the final mark. In nine sessions, with a peer teacher assignment twice, 11 points can be earned (7*1 point plus 2*2 points). Access to the final written test requires at least 5 points for active participation. Points from 6 on (until 11) are counted toward the overall final score, while each of those points counts twice, yielding 12 points (6*2). This is 12 % of the overall final score.

Active participation at all meetings is expected. Missed sessions may be replaced in another group. Attending at another group is advisable if this other group and the consultant agree, but this is not rewarded with points. In case of three or more sessions missed, students need to contact the coordinator and may gain an exception through the study counselor if they have a sound reason.[4]

CBCR Session Participation Points

[Gives information on how students are assessed during group meetings, see for more explanation Chap. 7. Make a distinction between points for students and points for peer teacher. Describe the criteria for receiving points/scores clearly.]

Active Participation During the Group Meetings: Students

The assessment of the participation occurs at the end of each meeting. The consultant indicates which students have actively participated, considering the following criteria[5]:

Students gain *1 point per meeting* for satisfactory participation. A student can receive 0 points for two reasons:

- Unsatisfactory participation in the discussion. Each student should participate in the discussion. A student who remains silent out of embarrassment or modesty is stimulated by the peer teachers or consultant, but must participate. *Silent presence is not enough.*
- Unsatisfactory preparation. From the active participation should show that there is a thorough preparation. Only with background knowledge a student can make a meaningful contribution. *It is not enough if the student wants to participate but doesn't give substantive contribution.* The latter doesn't mean to create an exam atmosphere, but it is important to properly prepare for each meeting.

Peer Teachers Roles

Peer teachers are expected to show a more extensive preparation than the students. The peer teachers must have a substantive performance at the meeting, which is especially reflected in the quality of justifying reports of the thinking steps in the

---

[4] Rules mentioned in this paragraph are used at the University Medical Center Utrecht, however, can be adapted to align with the local situation.

[5] Criteria and scores mentioned in this paragraph are used at the University Medical Center Utrecht, however, can be adapted to align with the local situation.

clinical process. They must demonstrate pathophysiological background knowledge and understanding of the clinical process.

Peer teachers can gain *up to 2 points per meeting*. The consultant will pay close attention to the way discussions are guided, to the peer teachers' additional background knowledge, and to the way they take leadership over the group. Scores are given as follows:

- 0 for poor preparation, no good leadership of the session
- 1 for moderate preparation, moderate leadership of the session
- 2 for good preparation, good leadership of the session

Each student must fulfill the peer teacher role twice. It is possible to earn a maximum of 1 bonus point by fulfilling the role of peer teacher for a third time to compensate for illness or absence at another meeting. There are never more than three peer teachers per meeting. The group as a whole is responsible for ensuring that there are at least two students functioning as a peer teacher at every meeting.

Disputes

We aim to provide good quality education by the consultants for the lessons. It is however possible that guidance or marking by the consultants leads to a dispute with a student. For any comments or disputes, we ask you kindly to contact the coordinator of the course [email address].

The CBCR Test

[In this paragraph students should be explained when the test will take place and what they can expect for the test. Examples of possible questions can be given here.]

The CBCR test is composed of questions that begin with a brief case description in which the age, sex, and the complaint with which the patients presents himself at the doctor are made clear. After this some additional information may be given and several questions follow.

The students are asked to choose the correct answer out of a table. The possible answers are displayed in a table, broken down by category: "diagnosis," "history features," "physical examination," "diagnostic test options," and "management." Sometimes there is asked for only one answer, sometimes for more.

A mock exam will be distributed a month before the test.

[Here example of test questions can be included. See for an example of the Utrecht CBCR test Chap. 7, Table 7.1].

Rules for Test Participation and Passing

[In this section the terms and conditions to participate in the test should be described. If students must have fulfilled certain conditions as minimal points for participation or minimal presence, this should be clarified here. Any regulations about possible compensation for missed classes can be described. Rules for passing the CBCR course need to be described.]

Rules for the Exam Retake

[Any rules and regulations for the exam retake should be clarified here.]

Rules for Repeaters

[Any rules and regulations for the repeaters should be clarified here.]

Open Access This chapter is licensed under the terms of the Creative Commons Attribution 4.0 International License (http://creativecommons.org/licenses/by/4.0/), which permits use, sharing, adaptation, distribution and reproduction in any medium or format, as long as you give appropriate credit to the original author(s) and the source, provide a link to the Creative Commons license and indicate if changes were made.

The images or other third party material in this chapter are included in the chapter's Creative Commons license, unless indicated otherwise in a credit line to the material. If material is not included in the chapter's Creative Commons license and your intended use is not permitted by statutory regulation or exceeds the permitted use, you will need to obtain permission directly from the copyright holder.

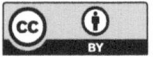

Appendix

Exemplary CBCR Case 1: A 17-Year-Old Girl with a Swelling in the Neck
Exemplary CBCR Case 2: A 68-Year-Old Man with Swollen Legs
Exemplary CBCR Case 3: A 47-Year-Old Woman with Fatigue
Exemplary CBCR Case 4: Two Patients with Hearing Loss

Appendix

Exemplary CBCR Case 1

A 17-Year-Old Girl with a Swelling in the Neck

Consultant Version

Designed and revised by many authors across many years at University Medical Center Utrecht. Translated and edited for this volume by Steven Durning MD PhD and Lieke van Imhoff MD.

Introduction

A swelling in the neck occurs frequently and can have different causes. In the pediatric population, this is often the result of an enlargement of one or more lymph nodes. Additional information obtained from a careful history and physical examination can help to provide the most likely diagnosis.

Objective of This CBCR Case

The student will identify the different causes of a swelling in the neck. The student will explain how to distinguish between these various disorders based on history, physical examination, and additional diagnostic testing. The student will discuss different treatment options and will be able to briefly summarize a case.

Preparation[1]

All students are to prepare questions 1–3 of the case using the given literature.
  Background literature for students

1. De Jongh et al. Diagnostiek van alledaagse klachten. Hoofdstuk 6: vergrote lymfeklieren. Houten: Bohn Stafleu van Loghum; 2011. p. 93–105

   Additional background literature for peer teachers

1. Velde van de CJH, Krieken JHJM, Mulder de PHM, Vermorken JB. Oncologie. Achtste herziene druk. Houten: Bohn Stafleu van Loghum; 2011. p. 581–96 [Dutch]
2. Lissauer T, Clayden G, editors. Illustrated textbook of Pediatrics. 4th edition. London: Elsevier; 2012. p. 371–73

---

[1] Preparation and assessment rules as used at UMC Utrecht – to be adapted to local requirements

Assessment

Students: Active participation in the session, 1 point; absent or present but not actively participating, 0 points.

Peer teachers: Excellent preparation and leadership of the session, 2 points; sufficient preparation and deficient leadership, 1 point; poor preparation and leadership, 0 points.

Suggested Time Schedule During the Session

Question 1–3	25 min
Question 4–5	20 min
Question 6–7	15 min
Question 8–9	20 min
Mini lecture	5 min
Question 10–11	20 min

Stage 1: Presentation of the Patient's Problem

You are a general practitioner (GP). Mr. Evans visits your office together with his 17-year-old daughter Emily. You know Emily as an insecure girl.

Mr. Evans tells you that Emily has a swelling in her neck for 6 weeks. Emily had a cold at the start of this period, so Mr. Evans was not worried at all. However, the swelling still exists and has become even more visible. Therefore, Mr. Evans insisted that his daughter visits your office.

Four months ago Emily consulted you because of a persistent cold. A chest X-ray was obtained because her father insisted: no abnormalities were seen. Against your own typical practice, you prescribed antibiotics. Now, Emily also suffers from itching. "Could she be allergic to those antibiotics doctor? All those medications, I do not like it," Mr. Evans says. During the whole consultation, Mr. Evans talks with you while Emily stares absently out of the window.

Question 1 What is the chief complaint of this patient? Can you identify the request for help?

Hints for Peer Teachers

Would the request for help[2] of the parents be the same as Emily's request for help? Do Emily's parents think of possible/specific causes of the swelling?

---

[2]The request for help is the underlying motive of a patient for visiting a doctor and the goal a patient wants to achieve with the visit.

Appendix

Is it likely that the itching is caused by antibiotics that were given 4 months ago, like Mr. Evans is thinking?

Background Information for the Consultant

The main complaint of this patient is a swelling in the neck, noticed 6 weeks ago.

The perception of Emily's parents plays a major role in their request for help. They are worried about their daughter. It is possible that they are considering Pfeiffer's disease, another infection or even a malignancy. It is important to find out their concerns about their daughter's complaints to assist your diagnostic and therapeutic decisions.

Emily's concerns are not clear yet: is she also worried about these symptoms? Does she want to know the cause of the swelling or does she just want to reassure her parents? She did not talk at all yet. She does not seem to be as worried as her father.

Emily also suffers from itching. Persistent itching *4 months* after taking antibiotics cannot be caused by a drug allergy. Drug reactions will usually subside after stopping the drug.

In infectious mononucleosis an itchy rash can occur when one is treated with amoxicillin, but it is also very unlikely this still persists after 4 months.

Question 2 Make an initial classification of possible causes of the main complaint

Hints for Peer Teachers

Try to structure the answers of the students. Make a table with different groups of conditions that can cause a swelling in the neck in the first column, such as infections. Also think about conditions other than the ones caused by lymphadenopathy.

How common are these different conditions? What is your differential diagnosis in this case?

	History		Physical examination		Additional investigations	
	For	*Against*	*For*	*Against*	*For*	*Against*
Lymphadenopathy						
Infections - Viral - Bacterial - Et cetera						
Other causes of a swelling in the neck						

Background Information for the Consultant

The goal of this table is to teach students how to perform analytic clinical reasoning. Let them think of examples of conditions in each group to improve their understanding of the concept. You can find the whole table in the appendix. The rest of the table will be filled in later during this session.

Students can experience difficulties with making a differential diagnosis. It can help to point out to structure causes by organ systems or main categories of illnesses.

The most common causes of enlarged lymph nodes are viral and bacterial infections. Also a malignancy is sometimes seen in lymphadenopathy (4 % in patients older than 40 years compared to 0.4 % in patients younger than 40 years). Hodgkin's lymphoma most commonly occurs between the age of 15 and 45 years and often starts with an enlarged cervical lymph node. Lymphatic leukemia does not typically present itself with an enlarged lymph node, but with general complaints. Systemic diseases are rare and it is extremely rare that enlarged lymph nodes are the first symptom. Lymphadenopathy as a side effect of medication is rare.

Lipomas and sebaceous cysts mainly occur in adults, and they are well distinguishable from a swollen lymph node on physical examination. Also a thyroid swelling is usually well distinguishable because of its localization centrally in the neck. A thyroglossal duct cyst is rare and is usually detected in childhood. A branchial cleft cyst might still present itself in young adulthood.

Question 3   What additional history questions can you ask to distinguish between the different possible causes?

Hints for Peer Teachers

Think of questions that will make diagnoses listed in the previous question more or less likely.

Let the students explain *why* they are asking a particular question: *how* can this question help discriminate between different diagnoses?

Try to structure the answers by dividing the questions into questions you want to ask about the swelling and questions for the full history or history of present illness.

Background Information for the Consultant

General questions are also part of history taking. The emphasis of this exercise is on the specific questions whose answers will influence the differential diagnosis.

Questions that can be useful:

- Is the swelling painful?
  Usually, swollen lymph nodes are not painful. Pain can be caused by inflammation. Painful nodes after drinking alcohol are described in Hodgkin's lymphoma.

Appendix

- Is there one swelling or are there more?
  It is important to differentiate between a solitary and a generalized swelling.
- Is the swelling (quickly) growing larger?
  Three to four weeks is a reasonable time period in accordance with a swollen lymph node due to infection. After this period further research needs to be done. A slow growth is suspected for malignancy.
- Does the patient have fever, night sweats, and/or weight loss? (B symptoms)
  These symptoms can be associated with malignancies or systemic diseases.
- Does the patient suffer from generalized itching?
- *Generalized itching can be associated with hematologic malignancies such as Hodgkin's lymphoma.*
- Did the patient visit a foreign country?
  This would make other causes of an infectious swelling more likely.
- Does the patient have pets?
  That you would have to think of cat-scratch disease (caused by the bacterium Bartonella henselae) or toxoplasmosis (caused by the protozoan Toxoplasma gondii, which is sometimes carried by cats in their feces).
- Does the patient use any drugs?
  Some antiepileptic drugs can cause lymphadenopathy as a very rare side effect.
- Questions that can help to reveal the request of help of Emily:
  Is Emily worried herself? Do the complaints influence her functioning? (e.g., bad sleeping because of the itching, fretting about the cause)

Stage 2: Results of History Taking
The swelling seems to have worsened over the last few weeks. Emily did not notice any rash or wounds. The last couple of weeks, she feels very tired and listless. She finds it hard to leave her bed. She did not measure her temperature, but wakes up often because of profuse sweating. Emily has missed a lot of school in the last few weeks. She does not know if she lost weight. She does not use any drugs besides the recent antibiotic therapy. Her cold is already over for a couple of weeks. Actually, she discovered the swelling in her neck afterward. She did not notice any swellings at other places in her body. Emily does not have any other complaints besides the swelling and the tiredness. There was no contact with cats and she never traveled outside Europe. Last year she was on holiday in France.

Question 4   Which components of the history taking help you to distinguish between the different groups of causes?

Hints for Peer Teachers

Discuss the different components of the history with the students. Let the students place the information from the handout in the table. If a diagnosis becomes more likely with certain information, place this information in the "for" box. If certain information makes a diagnosis less likely, place this information in the "against" box.

Background Information for the Consultant

It is a solitary swelling without a local or regional infection that could explain the swelling. The swelling has been there too long to be explained by the recent upper respiratory tract infection.

The symptoms of malaise and night sweats might suggest an underlying malignancy, as well as the possible growth of the swelling. These symptoms can also be seen in tuberculosis or HIV. A systemic disease is less likely because this is a solitary swelling.

Question 5   Which components of the physical examination should you perform? How can these examinations help to distinguish between the different conditions?

Hints for Peer Teachers

Students should decide which aspects of physical examination they want to perform. Let them explain how these examinations will help to distinguish between the different conditions.

Try to structure this question by dividing the physical examination into examination of the swelling and a general examination. Separate inspection, palpation, and auscultation.

Background Information for the Consultant

The physical examination of this patient will include the following:
Physical examination of the swelling:

- Distinguish between swollen lymph nodes and other swellings.
  If the swelling is located in an area where no lymph nodes are found, this distinction is easily made. Sebaceous cysts or inflamed sweat glands may occur, especially in the armpits and groin. These are identified by the fact that they are normally connected to the skin. Lipomas are deeper under the skin and normally larger than lymph nodes.

Appendix

- Examination of the lymph nodes: exact localization, consistency, size, freely movable, or fixed to underlying structures.
  Tender, mobile, painful lymph nodes typically represent inflammation from an infection. Hard, fixed, non-painful lymph nodes are suspicious for malignancy. In general 10 mm is considered the upper limit of normal nodes. The probability of a malignancy increases with the size of the node.
  Physical examination in general:
- Palpation of other lymph node stations (neck, groin, armpit)
  General swelling of lymph node stations throughout the body might indicate an infection (such as mononucleosis infectiosa or HIV), a systemic disease, or a non-Hodgkin's lymphoma.
- Examination of the ENT system
  To identify a possible focus of infection.
- Inspection of the skin
  Because of the itching, you should look for redness, evidence of scratching, or dry skin.

General measurements:

- Measuring temperature
  To identify a possible fever
- Measuring weight
  To monitor her weight

Stage 3: Results of Physical Examination
Emily is a pale, tired looking girl. Her temperature is 37.1°°C.

She now weighs 49 k and remembers she weighed 52 k 6 weeks ago. Her skin does not show redness or other abnormalities. Examination of the ears, nose, and throat shows no abnormalities either. You feel a hard, cervical lymph node located on the left lateral base of the neck, next to the sternocleidomastoid muscle. It is about 3–4 cm in diameter and freely movable from the skin but fixed to the underlying structures. The swelling is not painful. No abnormal lymph nodes are felt on the other lymph node stations.

Question 6 Which components of the physical examination help you to distinguish between the different conditions? What is the most likely diagnosis now?

Hints for Peer Teachers

Discuss the different components of the physical examination one by one with the students.

Let the students place the information from the handout in the table. If a diagnosis becomes more likely with certain information, place this information in the "for" box. If certain information makes a diagnosis less likely, place this information in the "against" box.

Now look at the entire table: what is the most likely diagnosis? Are there diagnoses you can exclude?

Background Information for the Consultant

The size of the lymph node (3–4 cm in diameter), and the fact that it is fixed to the underlying tissue, is suggestive for a malignancy. Also the weight loss supports this hypothesis.

Tuberculosis cannot be ruled out, but seems to be less likely in this young, native patient.

Question 7   Which diagnostic investigations need to be done to confirm or exclude remaining diagnoses?

Hints for Peer Teachers

Let the student think about laboratory and possible supplementary investigations. Keep in mind that the possibilities for you as a general practitioner are limited.

If students come up with multiple answers, let them choose what they really want to investigate and how this will help them to distinguish between diseases.

Background Information for the Consultant

Blood tests and chest X-ray should be performed in this patient. The blood tests will include a complete blood count with differential and an erythrocyte sedimentation rate (ESR). Also a serological test for EBV might be performed. It is important to realize that normal laboratory values sometimes cannot rule out the beginning of a serious condition. The chest X-ray is useful to identify a possible widened mediastinum and/or findings consistent with tuberculosis.

Regardless of the lab results, the GP will consult the pediatrician, given the seriousness of the pathology in the differential diagnosis. In the hospital further diagnostic investigations may be carried out, depending on the results of the blood test and chest X-ray.

Appendix

Stage 4: Results of Diagnostic Tests
You decide to send Emily to the laboratory for a blood test. A chest X-ray will be performed as well. You agree with Emily and her parents that they will come back the next day after a few days to discuss the results. The laboratory results are as follows:

Hemoglobin	*7.4 mmol/L*	*(Normal range: 7.4–9.6 mmol/L, in women)*
Leukocytes	*6.4 × 10^9/L Differential without abnormalities*	*(Normal range: 4.0–10.0 × 10^9/L)*
Platelets	*234 × 10^9/L*	*(Normal range: 150–400 × 10^9/L)*
ESR	*65 mm/h*	*(Normal range: 2–24 mm/h, in women)*
EBV serological test	*Negative*	

You look at the chest X-ray and compare it with that of 4 months ago

Chest X-ray 4 months ago *Current chest X-ray*

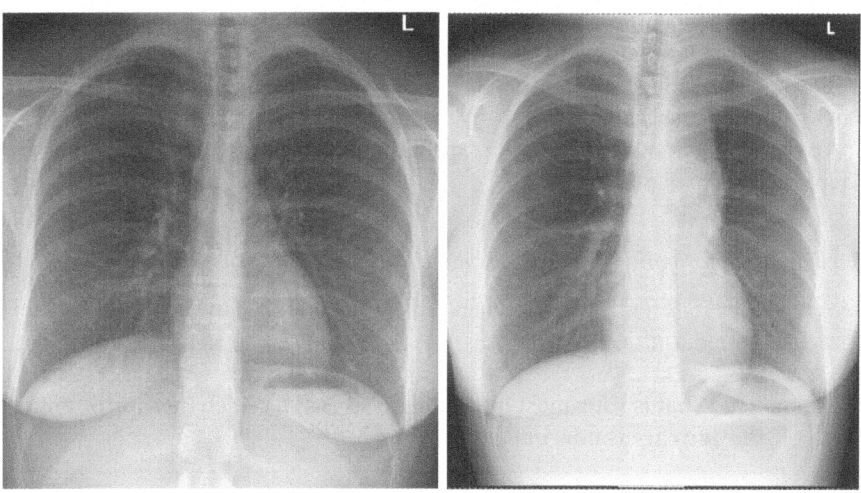

Question 8   What do you see on the chest X-ray?

Hints for Peer Teachers

Let the students describe both X-rays systematically starting with the quality of the X-ray and all the structures and finishing with the abnormalities.

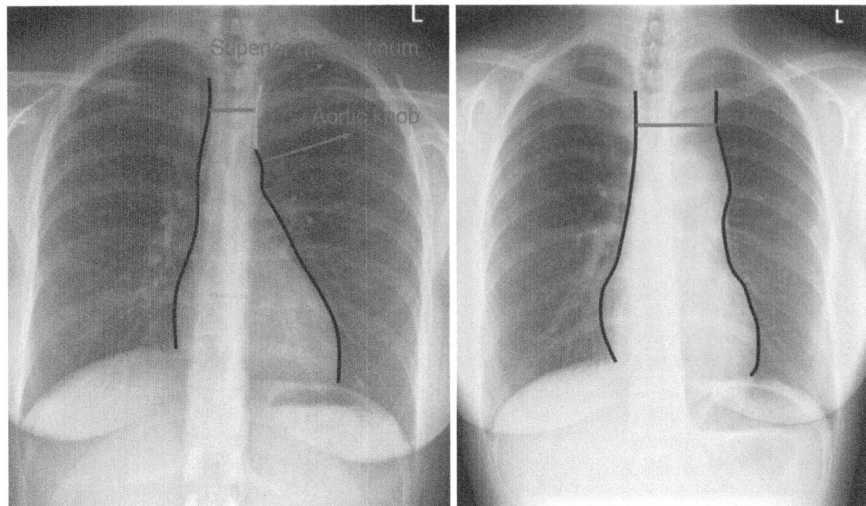

The chest X-ray on the left was made 4 months ago when Emily had complaints of cough and fever. This image does not show any abnormalities.

The chest X-ray on the right reveals a widening of the superior mediastinum. You can see a significant difference from the previous chest X-ray. In the next image, the width of the mediastinum is indicated by a red line. Because of this widening, the aortic knob is no longer recognizable. The heart has a normal shape and size. The lungs show no abnormalities.

The widening of the superior mediastinum is most likely caused by lymphadenopathy.

Background Information for the Consultant

See the suggestions for the peer teachers. Take a good look at the images before the session is started.

Question 9   What is your most likely diagnosis now? Which therapy or policy for care is now indicated?

Hints for Peer Teachers

Discuss both the lab results and the chest X-ray with the students. Let them place the results in the table again.

The chest radiograph is the most notable finding. A malignancy is likely. The lymphadenopathy might also be caused by tuberculosis, but no typical infiltrates are seen on the X-ray, and the history does not mention any travel to endemic areas or contact with infected people.

Appendix

Which type of malignancy is the most likely? Which diagnostic investigations need to be done? Do you have to refer Emily to a medical specialist?

Background Information for the Consultant

Emily most likely has a malignant lymphoma, presumably Hodgkin's disease because of her age. Hodgkin's disease most commonly occurs in early adulthood and in late adulthood (after age of 55). However, a non-Hodgkin's lymphoma can also be the cause.

Emily should be referred to a pediatric hematologist for further investigation and treatment. To be sure of the diagnosis, an excisional biopsy of the lymph node is necessary. Fine needle aspiration (FNA) biopsy is not enough to diagnose Hodgkin's disease, because it normally does not provide enough tissue.

Also additional imaging evaluation is needed to evaluate the lymphatic system. A CT scan will be made. In addition, a PET scan or an integrated PET-CT scan can be performed. Finally, a bone marrow biopsy should be considered to identify possible marrow involvement. This is rare in Hodgkin's disease. The stage of the disease can be determined after all these diagnostic tests are performed.

Stage 5: Results of Therapeutic Management
You refer Emily to a pediatrician who performs additional testing. On the basis of a biopsy and a PET-CT scan, the diagnosis Hodgkin's lymphoma stage IIB is made (CT scan of the chest, suspected lymphoma in the mediastinum; abdominal CT scan, no abnormalities; bone marrow biopsy, no abnormalities). Emily is being treated with chemotherapy. She tolerates this fairly well. Side effects she has experienced are hair loss and nausea on the day of therapy. Once she gets a fever with leukopenia, she is admitted to receive intravenous antibiotics.

Six months after being diagnosed, she is completely cancer-free. According to the attending pediatric hematologist, her prognosis is favorable; she estimates her chance of complete cure at more than 90 %.

Mini lecture: A short presentation is given by one of the peer teachers

Hints for Peer Teachers

Now one of the peer teachers gives a mini lecture (max 5 min, max five slides). The purpose of this lecture is to explain briefly and clearly about Hodgkin's lymphoma to your fellow students. It is certainly not the intention to give a complete and detailed overview of the disease.

Answer the following questions in this lecture:

- What is the incidence of Hodgkin's lymphoma and at what age does the disease occurs mainly?
- What is the pathophysiology of the disease?
- What is, broadly, the difference between Hodgkin's and non-Hodgkin's lymphoma?
- What is the treatment (broadly, no specific details about types of chemotherapy and other drugs are needed)?
- What is the prognosis?

Question 10 One of the students from the group summarizes the whole case chronologically in a few minutes

Hints for Peer Teachers

If necessary, you can help the students to summarize using the following format:

During the office hour I saw a ... year old man/woman with complaints of ... Patient has ..... as relevant prehistory. Relevant medication is.....

The major problem during history taking is .... During the physical examination, I saw ..... Additional test showed ... (special findings or negative findings). In conclusion, I saw a ... year old man/woman with probably ..... (working diagnosis) for which I want to start ... (additional testing or policy). In the differential diagnosis I still consider.....

Question 11 Now suppose Emily reveals a different history. Which diagnoses are most likely?

1. A 17-year-old girl has enlarged lymph nodes in her neck and throat pain. On physical examination you find painful, enlarged lymph nodes on both sides and a red pharynx with enlarged tonsils with debris.
2. A 17-year-old girl has enlarged lymph nodes in her neck, throat pain, and since 2 days an itchy rash. She is already treated with antibiotics because it was thought to be a bacterial tonsillitis. On physical examination you find painful, enlarged lymph nodes on both sides. The liver edge is palpable about 2 cm below the right costal margin.
3. A 17-year-old girl, fled with her family from Eritrea a few years ago, presents with a solitary enlarged lymph node in her neck. She lost 4 kg in a month and suffers from night sweats.
4. A 17-year-old girl has swellings in her neck, which are mobile when swallowing. She has complaints of palpitations, hair loss, and profuse sweating.

Appendix

Hints for Peer Teachers

This exercise is a good test to see whether the students master the subject. You can use the completed table, which will give you a lot of information. It is about pointing out the most likely diagnosis. On basis of the limited information given, other diagnoses cannot be excluded.

Background Information for the Consultant

1. Reactive lymphadenopathy on the basis of a tonsillitis (upper respiratory tract infection) is the most likely diagnosis. Tonsillitis is usually caused by a viral infection. Some cases can also be caused by a bacterial infection, typically a group A streptococcus.
2. Mononucleosis (an EBV infection) is now more likely, because of the palpable liver edge. The skin rash fits with a viral infection but can also be caused by antibiotic use in EBV infection.
3. The swelling in combination with night sweats and weight loss are alarming symptoms. Tuberculosis is high in the differential diagnosis because of her origin. Another tropical infection or malignant lymphoma cannot be excluded.
4. The symptoms best fit with hyperthyroidism. This may be caused by a toxic multinodular goiter, given the fact different swellings are present. Let the students realize that a swelling can also be caused by something other than lymphadenopathy.

Appendix

	History		Physical examination		Diagnostic investigations	
	For	Against	For	Against	Pro	Against
Lymphadenopathy						
Infections						
Reaction to local infection like tonsillitis	Age, night sweats (TBC)	No signs of local infection, no cats (against cat-scratch disease, toxoplasmosis), no tropical countries (against parasitic, TBC)	Weight loss (TBC)	Non-painful, fixed to underlying structures, no abnormalities in ENT area	Increased ESR	No lymphocytosis, EBV negative (against EBV)
Viral (e.g., EBV, CMV)						
Bacterial (e.g., TBC, cat-scratch disease)						
Parasitic (e.g., toxoplasmosis)						
Fungal						
Malignancy						
Drainage local primary tumor	Age (lymphoma), itching, night sweats, malaise, growth of swelling	Age (against metastasis)	Non-painful, weight loss, hard consistency, fixed to underlying structures		Widened mediastinum on chest X-ray (most likely caused by lymphadenopathy), increased ESR	
Lymphoma (Hodgkin/non-Hodgkin)						
Lymphatic leukemia						
Metastasis of other tumor (e.g., head and neck tumor)						

Systemic disease	Malaise	Solitary swelling				
SLE						
Sarcoidosis						
Drugs		No drugs use, no other complaints (rash, arthralgia)				
Phenytoin						
Carbamazepine						
Other causes of a swelling in the neck						
Thyroid swelling	Additional complaints		Weight loss	Location of the swelling		
Solitary nodule						
Multinodular						
Struma						
(Sub)cutaneous swelling		Age, itching, malaise, night sweats		Not fixed to the skin		
Lipoma						
Sebaceous cyst						
Congenital		Recent onset of swelling, additional complaints				
Thyroglossal duct cyst						
Branchial cleft cyst						

Appendix 151

Exemplary CBCR Case 2

A 68-Year-Old Man with Swollen Legs

Consultant Version

Designed by Gaiane Simonia, M.D. Ph.D., at Tbilisi State Medical University and edited for this volume by Maria van Loon M.D.

Introduction

A common challenge for primary care physicians is to determine the cause and to find an effective treatment for patients with a swollen leg or both legs swollen. A variety of clinical conditions, ranging from the benign to the potentially life-threatening, is associated with the development of peripheral edema. These include common conditions such as heart failure, liver cirrhosis, and nephrotic syndrome, as well as local leg swelling due to deep vein thrombosis, use of certain medications, or represent idiopathic edema. A systematic approach to the patient with swollen lower extremities allows for prompt and cost-effective diagnosis and treatment.

Objective of This CBCR Case

Ability to determine causes of peripheral edema (swelling of legs) and to learn general principles of management of cardiac edema in the initial stages of heart failure.

Preparation[3]

All students should prepare questions 1–5 of the case at home by using the given literature.

Background Literature for Students

- Harrison's Principles of Internal Medicine: Volumes 1 and 2, 18th Edition, p. 290
- Kumar V, Abbas AK, Aster JC. *Robbins and Cotran Pathologic Basis of Disease*, 8th ed. Elsevier Saunders, Philadelphia 2010, Chapter 4. Hemodynamic disorders, Thromboembolic disease, and Shock. Edema
- Ferri: Ferri's Clinical Advisor 2012, 1st ed

---

[3] Preparation and assessment rules as used at TSMU – to be adapted to local requirements

Additional Background Literature for Peer Teachers

- Fly JW, Osheroff JA, Chambliss ML, Ebel MH. Approach to leg edema of unclear etiology. *Journal of the American Board of Family Medicine* 2006;19:148–160
- Ramanathan M. Idiopathic Edema: A Lesson in Differential Diagnosis. *Medical Journal of Malaysia*. 1994;49:285–288
- Beth E. Schroth, Evaluation and management of peripheral edema. *Journal of the American Academy of Physician Assistants*. 2005;18:29–34
- Skorecki K, Chertow GM, Marsden PA, Taal MW, Yu ASL. *Brenner and Rector's* The *Kidney*. Philadelphia, PA: WB Saunders 2011, 9 ed, p. 1894

Assessment

Students: Active participation in the session, 1 point; absent or present but not actively participating, 0 points

Peer teachers: Excellent preparation and leadership of the session, 2 points; sufficient preparation and deficient leadership, 1 point; poor preparation and leadership, 0 points.

Proposed Time Schedule

Stage I
Question 1   5 min
Question 2   10 min
Question 3   10 min
Question 4   10 min
Question 5   5 min

Stage II
  Handout 1
Question 6   10 min
Question 7   5 min
Question 8   10 min
  Mini lecture: 10 min

Stage III
  Handout 2
Question 9:   10 min
Question 10   10 min
Summary: 10 min

Appendix

> **Stage 1: Presentation of the Patient's Problem**
> Mr. Nicholas Giorgadze, a 68-year-sold male, comes to your GP office with a 6-month history of progressive fatigue, dizziness, and swelling of legs. During this period he noticed he has gained some weight. He also noticed gradually reduced urine volume and swelling of legs, mostly in the evening or after a prolonged sitting position. Mr. Giorgadze is a writer and usually works with his PC until late in the evening, but he never developed swollen legs before.

Question 1 Based on the case presentation, what could be the cause of the swelling of the legs, and are there any predisposing factors of peripheral edema?

Hints for Peer Teachers

Students should clarify whether edema occurs in the morning and in the evening or persists the whole day. Since leg edema might be due to continuous sitting as well, students should ask about excreted urine volume.

Background Information for the Consultant

Usually peripheral edema follows sodium retention and decrease in diuresis. Initially it occurs in the evening and/or after prolonged sitting position.

Question 2 Based on the history, what is the most likely problem of the patient?

Hints for Peer Teachers

Based on the pathogenesis of different types of edema, students have to clarify:

- Which type of edema does the patient have (generalized vs. local, uni- or bilateral)?
- What is the *duration* of the edema (acute [72 h] vs. chronic)?

Background Information for the Consultant

Peripheral edema is a common problem. A wide range of systemic and regional disorders can result in fluid retention in the peripheries. Identification of cardiac causes of leg swelling is based on the consideration and exclusion of all other possible causes. It is important that students can differentiate generalized and local edema of the legs. They need to use their knowledge of the pathogenesis of edema and possible causes of leg swelling.

The patient presented in this case highlights some of the salient features of the cardiac edema (appearance of leg swelling in the evening, reduced urine volume) although it should be noted that bilateral leg edema is a relatively nonspecific symptom of heart failure (compared to dyspnea, orthopnea, etc.); in elderly persons (having mostly sedentary lifestyle) it might reflect peripheral rather than cardiac causes.

Question 3   Make an initial classification of possible causes of edema that can lead to leg swelling.

Hints for Peer Teachers

Create a table of different groups of conditions that can lead to edema. Consider organ systems or medications that can cause leg swelling.

	Likely	Less likely	Not very likely
Hypothesis 1			
Hypothesis 2			
Hypothesis 3			
Hypothesis 4			
Hypothesis 5			
Hypothesis 6			
Hypothesis 7			
Hypothesis 8			

Background Information for the Consultant

Evaluation of the patient with peripheral edema needs a multisystem approach. Of particular importance is to exclude organ system dysfunction, especially cardiac, liver, and renal dysfunction. Local causes such as venous insufficiency and lymphedema, as well as medication-induced leg swelling, should also be considered. Based on aforementioned, it is recommended to draw the following type of grid table:

Possible causes	Likely	Less likely	Not very likely
Cardiac failure			
Liver cirrhosis			
Nephrotic syndrome			
Venous insufficiency			
Lymphedema			
Medications			
Pulmonary hypertension			
Idiopathic edema			

Appendix

Question 4 Discuss pathophysiological mechanisms of leg swelling formation, related to the possible causes listed above.

Hints for Peer Teachers

Students should draw a table with lists of possible pathophysiological mechanisms leading to edema.

Pathophysiological mechanisms of peripheral edema
1
2
3
4
5

Background Information for the Consultant

Students should be able to consider pathophysiological features of edema due to different causative conditions.

Pathophysiological mechanisms of peripheral edema
1. Decreased oncotic pressure
2. Increased hydrostatic pressure
3. Activation of RAAS and natriuretic system
4. Increased capillary permeability
5. Lymphatic obstruction
6. Inflammation and hypercoagulation

Question 5 What additional history questions should you ask to proceed in identifying the cause of edema?

Hints for Peer Teachers

Questions should help to identify causative factors for leg edema. Therefore students should justify their questions – how can they lead to the right diagnosis?

The most common questions that students might ask are:

- How long does the edema exist?
- Is the edema uni- or bilateral?
- Is the edema localized only in legs or in other parts of the body as well?
- Is it pitting edema?
- Is the edema painful?
- What color has the skin locally over the edema?

- Does the edema still persist in the morning?
- Is the patient obese?
- Does the patient suffer from dyspnea?
- Does he experience fatigue?
- Does the patient consume salty meal?
- Does he have nocturia?

Background Information for the Consultant

The most common questions might be the following:

- What is the *duration* of the edema (<72 h/acute or chronic). If the onset is acute, deep vein thrombosis should be ruled out at first. In this case this question is not applicable, because the patient noticed that the leg edema appeared appr. 6 months ago.
- Is the edema *uni-* or *bilateral?* If unilateral, is there a history of pelvic/abdominal neoplasm (to exclude edema due to compression).
- *Pitting* or *non-pitting* leg edema? Edema caused by venous insufficiency or systemic diseases is pitting (when the skin over edema can be temporarily indented when pressed), while non-pitting edema is usually a sign of lymphedema or myxedema.
- Is the edema *painful?* Deep vein thrombosis and reflex sympathetic dystrophy are usually painful. Chronic venous insufficiency can cause low-grade aching. Lymphedema is usually painless.
- Is there a history of *systemic disease* (heart, liver, or kidney disease)?
- Does the swelling *improve overnight?* (Venous/dependent edema is more likely than lymphedema to reduce/disappear overnight.)
- What *medicines* are being taken? Certain drugs (calcium channel blockers, NSAIDs, steroids, estrogens, etc.) may cause swelling of legs.
- Is there a history consistent to *sleep apnea?* Sleep apnea can cause pulmonary hypertension which is a common cause of leg edema. Suspicious signs for sleep apnea are loud snoring, daytime somnolence, or a neck circumference more than 17 in.
- Does the patient experience *dyspnea* (paroxysmal nocturnal dyspnea, dyspnea on physical exertion or during rest): the most specific initial clinical sign of heart failure is *paroxysmal nocturnal dyspnea* that relieves by sitting or standing (*orthopnea*); further progression of heart failure is characterized by dyspnea appearing during physical stress; occurrence of dyspnea during rest indicates a severe stage of heart failure.
- Usually congestive heart failure is accompanied by *nocturia* (excessive urination at night); however nocturia is not a specific sign for heart failure; it might appear in renal failure as well as in physiological aging.

Appendix

Handout is shown on the screen and read out.

> **Stage 2: Results of History Taking**
> During history taking Mr. Giorgadze tells you that he has approximately a 6-year history of mild hypertension. However he did not take antihypertensive drugs regularly (he takes hydrochlorothiazide only during episodes of headache). His apartment is on the third floor. Normally he doesn't use the elevator, but recently he started using it because he felt short of breath while climbing the stairs. Mr. Giorgadze is used to consume salty meals.

Question 6   What diagnoses are most likely now?

Hints for Peer Teachers

Peer teacher draws a grid table on the flip chart to facilitate the formulation of proper questions (this can be done before the session, but should be revealed only at this moment). Insert with the student the data from the history in the table. Which diagnoses appear most likely now?

DD	HF	LC	NS	VI	Lymph	Drugs	PH	IE
1. Leg edema> 72 h (during appr. 6 months)								
2. Painless swelling								
3. Bilateral								
4. Improves at night								
5. Shortness of breath on exertion								
6. History of hypertension								
7. Reduced urine volume								
8. Consuming salty meals								

HF heart failure, *LC* liver cirrhosis, *NS* nephrotic syndrome, *VI* venous insufficiency, *PH* pulmonary hypertension, *IE* idiopathic edema

Background Information for the Consultant.

DD	HF	LC	NS	VI	Lymph.	Drugs	PH	IE
1. Leg edema> 72 h (appr. 6 months)	+	+	+	+	+	+	+	+
2. Painless swelling	+	+	+	+	+	+	+	+
3. Bilateral	+	+	+	+	+	+	+	+
4. Pitting	+	+	+	+	−	+	+	+
5. Improves at night	+	−	−	+	−	−	−	−
6. Shortness of breath on exertion	+	−	−	−	−	−	−	−
7. History of hypertension	+	−	−	−	−	−	−	−
8. Reduced urine volume	+	+	+	−	−	−	−	−
9. Consuming salty meals	+	+	+	−	−	−	−	−

HF heart failure, *LC* liver cirrhosis, *NS* nephrotic syndrome, *VI* venous insufficiency, *PH* pulmonary hypertension, *IE* idiopathic edema

Currently, among causative conditions heart failure is most likely.

Possible causes	Likely	Less likely	Not very likely
Cardiac failure	√		
Liver cirrhosis		√	
Nephrotic syndrome		√	
Venous insufficiency		√	
Lymphedema			√
Medications			√
Pulmonary hypertension			√
Idiopathic edema			√

Question 7   Which components of the physical examination should you perform? How can these examinations help to distinguish between different conditions leading to edema of the legs?

Hints for Peer Teachers

Students should decide which specific types of physical examination they want to perform (using inspection, palpation, percussion, and auscultation).

Background Information for the Consultant

Clinical evaluation of the patient should include the following:

Vital signs: Blood pressure, heart rate, respiratory rate, and jugular venous pressure are important features to come to the right diagnosis (i.e., low blood pressure is often seen in nephrotic syndrome or liver cirrhosis, while high blood pressure might indicate arterial hypertension as a cause of heart failure). Tachycardia may be a sign of heart failure to compensate the low stroke volume. Irregular, weak thread pulse or pulsus alternans is often associated with decreased left ventricular function. Increased respiratory rate is a very important indicator of dyspnea, especially at rest.

Inspection: Skin redness over the legs mostly indicates acute venous inflammation and thrombosis. Brown skin of the lower swollen legs is consistent with chronic venous insufficiency. Findings of heart failure (cyanosis, jugular venous distension, orthopnea), liver disease (spider hemangiomas, jaundice, dilated collateral veins on the abdomen – "caput medusa" – palmar erythema), and renal diseases (i.e., paleness due to severe anemia) may be very helpful in detecting a systemic cause.

Palpation and percussion: Palpation of the skin over swollen legs helps to reveal tenderness (i.e., in deep vein thrombosis or thrombophlebitis, while lymphedema usually is not accompanied by pain on palpation) and to differentiate pitting from non-pitting edema. Lymphedema is characterized by inability to pinch a fold of skin on the dorsum of the foot at the base of the second toe (Kaposi-Stemmer sign). In heart failure, palpation and percussion can reveal displacement of the point of maximal pulsation of the left ventricle and can be a sign of cardiomegaly. Using palpation and percussion, accumulation of fluid in abdominal (shifting dullness) and pleural cavities (dullness over lung bases) can be found in patients with generalized edema. The key component of the differential diagnosis in edematous patients is the evaluation of liver size by palpation and percussion. Hepatomegaly may occur in right ventricular heart failure as well as in liver cirrhosis. Also the presence of hepatojugular reflux can be a useful test (applying moderate pressure on the abdomen above the liver area) in patients with right-sided heart failure.

Auscultation: The most specific auscultation finding in heart failure is appearance of S3 which is indicative of high left ventricular dysfunction. In patients with diastolic heart failure, S4 heart sound can be revealed. Systolic and/or diastolic murmurs can provide information on the cause of heart failure. Pulmonary congestion is confirmed by audible rales and pleural effusion in severe cases.

Idiopathic edema can be diagnosed in young women without further testing if there is no reason to suspect another etiology, based on history and physical examination.

Question 8 **What diagnostic tests should you perform? Try to list tests that could reveal a specific disease related to peripheral edema.**

Hints for Peer Teachers

Since the cause of bilateral leg edema is multifactorial, a number of diagnostic tests (both biochemical and instrumental) should be performed to make the correct diagnosis.

Try to list blood tests that could reveal a specific disease related to peripheral edema. Also think of other diagnostic test that can help to distinguish between diagnoses such as radiological or noninvasive tests. How can a test result help you to rule in or out a specific diagnosis?

Background Information for Consultant

As the first step, the following laboratory tests will help to rule out systemic diseases as a causative factor of leg swelling: complete blood count, urinalysis, electrolytes (plasma levels of potassium and sodium), and creatinine, blood sugar, albumin, and bilirubin levels.

Patients who may have a cardiac etiology should have an electrocardiogram, echocardiogram, and chest radiograph. Dyspneic patients should have a brain natriuretic peptide (BNP) determination to help to detect heart failure. The BNP is considered to be the most helpful biomarker for ruling out (rather than ruling in) heart failure because of high (90 %) sensitivity.

Patients with possible nephrotic syndrome should have serum lipids determined in addition to the basic laboratory studies listed above. Patients with suggested liver cirrhosis should be additionally tested for certain serum enzymes (ALT, AST, alkaline phosphatase) and referred for noninvasive (ultrasonography, CT) and invasive (liver biopsy) investigations.

To exclude chronic venous insufficiency, a number of diagnostic investigations (ambulatory venous pressure monitoring, venous Duplex imaging, plethysmography) should be performed.

Mini lecture **After Question 8 one of peer teachers gives a mini lecture on specific diagnostic tests related to the differential diagnosis of peripheral edema**

Hints for Peer Teachers

Peripheral edema has multiple causes and is particularly nonspecific. Therefore, besides less objective and less reproducible signs (such as displacement of the apical pulsation, appearance of S3 or S4), a number of biochemical and instrumental tests are needed to clarify the diagnosis.

The mini lecture should summarize the information on specific diagnostic tests (biochemical, instrumental, and invasive) recommended to conduct for a proper differential diagnosis of peripheral edema indicating test specificity. It is important to show which tests are relevant for each of aforementioned suggested causative condition.

The presentation will facilitate the interpretation of the results of the diagnostic tests by students during stage III.

The mini lecture is meant to provide the students with information they can directly apply in the continuation of the case. Peer teachers should therefore make sure that the information in the mini lecture is directly applicable (i.e., explanation about pathophysiology or pros and cons of certain diagnostics). The goal of the mini lecture is not to have peer teachers comprehensively review a large topic. The purpose is not that of an examination to investigate how much this student knows; rather the mini lecture should provide all students with helpful background information and to stimulate their understanding of the case: this is true peer teaching. Peer teachers should be selective in what they present, as the presentation should never take longer than 10 min and usually much shorter.

Background Information for the Consultant

The background information may be more extensive than what the peer teachers are going to tell.

Briefly, a mini lecture should be given on the sequence of the physical examination and additional instrumental and lab tests in accordance to the following issues:

Systemic evaluation (biochemical tests):

- CBC
- Urinalysis
- Electrolytes
- Creatinine
- Blood glucose

- Bilirubin
- Albumin
- Lipids

Specific indications:

- Heart failure: ECG, echocardiography, plasma BNP level, chest X-ray
- Liver cirrhosis: ALT, AST, bilirubin, alkaline phosphatase, prothrombin time, serum albumin, ultrasonography, liver biopsy
- Nephrotic syndrome: serum albumin, urinalysis, creatinine, serum lipids
- Lymphedema: abdominal/pelvic CT scan (to exclude malignancy)
- Chronic venous insufficiency (ambulatory venous pressure monitoring, venous Duplex imaging, plethysmography)

Peer teachers should clarify the diagnostic route for each suspected pathological condition emphasizing significance and specificity of each test in the context of swollen legs.

In patients with swollen legs, CBC (complete blood analysis) data might indicate certain conditions. Leukocytosis and redness and tenderness of legs are suspicious for deep venous thrombosis, while anemia is more characteristic for chronic kidney disease.

Hypoalbuminemia (normal range 3.5–5.5 g/dl or 35–55 g/l, or 50 %–60 % of blood plasma proteins) usually appears in patients with nephrotic syndrome or liver cirrhosis. Routine urinalysis and plasma level of lipids could help to distinguish these two clinical conditions: heavy proteinuria, hypoalbuminemia, and hyperlipidemia (total cholesterol >10 mmol/l); elevated plasma level of creatinine (normal range 0.6–1.3 mg/dl or 53–115 mcmol/l) confirms renal pathology (nephrotic syndrome). If these changes are accompanied by hyperglycemia, nephrotic syndrome might be the result of diabetic nephropathy. Hyperbilirubinemia (normal range 0.2–1.2 mg/dL) and hypoalbuminemia most probably might be due to liver cirrhosis. Hypokalemia (normal range 3.5–5 mml/l) and hyponatremia (normal range 135–145 mmol/l) might be related to adverse effects of diuretics used in edematous states and lead to exacerbation of causative conditions.

Despite the significance of aforementioned tests, additional, more specific diagnostic tools are needed to confirm the final diagnosis and identification of the only condition that caused swollen legs. The following specific diagnostic tests are recommended for the suggested condition:

Heart failure; brain natriuretic peptide (BNP) is currently considered as the most specific (about 90 %) biomarker for heart failure. Chest X-ray may reveal cardiomegaly and pleural effusions; ECG may indicate the cause (myocardial infarction, ventricular hypertrophy, etc.). Echocardiography is more specific and may indicate the cause and confirm the presence of systolic or diastolic left ventricular dysfunction.

Liver cirrhosis: The most specific invasive diagnostic tool for liver cirrhosis is liver biopsy; however other noninvasive tests are also recommended: AST and ALT enzymes (although they are not specific). Liver ultrasound + Duplex may show liver size, focal lesions, and ascites; MRI (magnetic resonance imaging) can quantify the severity of cirrhosis and is considered a very useful test for estimating stage and prognosis of liver cirrhosis.

Nephrotic syndrome: Renal biopsy is the most specific invasive diagnostic test; however its use is limited. A less specific but widely used noninvasive diagnostic test is renal ultrasound (detects size, shape, and location of kidneys).

Lymphedema: Diagnosis of leg lymphedema is usually obvious from physical examination. Additional tests are indicated when secondary lymphedema is suspected. CT and MRI can identify sites of lymphatic obstruction; radionuclide lymphoscintigraphy can identify lymphatic hypoplasia or sluggish flow.

Chronic venous insufficiency: Venous Duplex imaging is a well-established rather specific method for the diagnosis of chronic venous insufficiency to assess its etiology and severity. Ambulatory venous pressure monitoring is considered an invasive gold standard in assessing the efficiency of the leg's musculovenous pump. The technique involves insertion of a needle into the pedal vein with connection to a pressure transducer. A less specific test is plethysmography, a noninvasive diagnostic tool that quantifies the physiologic components of chronic venous disease including chronic obstruction, valvular reflux, poor calf muscle pump function, and venous hypertension.

Handout is shown on the screen and read out loud.

Stage 3: Results of Physical Examination and Diagnostic Testsa
On physical examination the patient's blood pressure is 165/92 mm Hg with pulse 78 bpm, regular. His weight is 78 kg, height 172 cm. The jugular venous pressure (JVP) is not elevated. Auscultation of the lungs reveals dullness to percussion and rales at both lung bases. Auscultation of the heart revealed diminished S1; S3 is heard at the apex. The respiratory rate is 26 breaths/min. The liver and spleen are not enlarged and have no signs of ascites.

Laboratory evaluations including urinalysis, complete blood counts, erythrocyte sedimentation rate, fasting and postprandial blood sugar, and liver function tests were normal. Lipid profile showed hypercholesterolemia (total cholesterol 279 mg/dl (optimal <200 mg/dl; 200–239 mg/dl, borderline high; >240 mg/dl, high), elevated LDL 185 mg/dl (normal 100–129 mg/dl; 130–159 mg/dl, borderline high; >160 mg/dl, high), triglycerides 20 mg/dl (optimal <100 mg/dl; 101–150 mg/dl, normal; 151–199 mg/dl, borderline; >200 mg/dl, high).

ECG showed left ventricular hypertrophy, echocardiography revealed diastolic dysfunction of the left ventricle, while EF was normal (56 %, normal range 55–70 %). BNP appeared to be elevated (136 pg/ml, normal range 0–100 pg/ml) suggesting an early stage of heart failure.

Appendix

Question 9   What do the results of the physical examination and laboratory and diagnostic tests show? What is your diagnosis now?

Hints for Peer Teachers

Based on the results of patient's examination and diagnostic tests, students should discuss and decide which conditions might be ruled out and what the final diagnosis is now. Try to assess the significance of the performed diagnostic tests, and identify the most specific and helpful tests.

Try to be as precise as possible in making the diagnosis.

Background Information for the Consultant

Patient's swollen legs are the result of heart failure which is confirmed by rales in the lungs, elevated BNP in the blood plasma, evidence of diastolic failure, and hypertrophy of the left ventricle on echocardiography. The most specific test confirming heart failure is elevated plasma level of BNP. Noteworthy that this time the leg edema was not induced by right ventricular failure (JVP is normal, there is no congestion in the liver, etc.); swelling developed as a result of early activation of sodium-retaining neurohumoral factors; it was shown that in some patients, leg edema might develop already in the initial stages of heart failure. Heart failure in this case is the consequence of noncontrolled long-lasting arterial hypertension. Leg edema did not develop due to taking edema-causing medicines, since the patient is taking only hydrochlorothiazide.

Question 10   What is the treatment and prognosis for this patient?

Hints for Peer Teachers

Optimal management of this case should be based on treatment (non-pharmacological and medication) of the primary cause of heart failure, taking into account the type of cardiac dysfunction (systolic vs. diastolic), a proper diet, and physical activity. Based on the stage of heart failure, the chance of reversibility and the prognosis of the course of disease should be proposed. Taking into consideration that the patient has diastolic heart failure, what non-pharmacological approaches exist to increase end-diastolic volume of the left ventricle? (i.e., compressing stockings, although their efficacy to prevent further progression has not been shown yet).

Background Information for the Consultant

Non-pharmacological treatment of heart failure implies lifestyle modifications such as salt restriction (2–3 g/day), regular moderate exercise, and correction of modifiable underlying conditions (proper diet, weight loss in obesity, cessation of smoking). It was shown that compressing stockings increased end-diastolic volume in some patients with diastolic dysfunction although their efficacy to prevent further progression has not been proven yet.

Pharmacological treatment of heart failure, in great extent, depends on the type of left ventricular dysfunction. In systolic dysfunction diuretics, ACE (angiotensin-converting enzyme) inhibitors, ARBs (angiotensin receptor blockers), and beta-blockers are recommended.

In diastolic heart failure, less drugs have been adequately studied. However, ACE inhibitors, ARBs, and beta-blockers are generally used. The use of an implantable cardioverter-defibrillator (ICD) or cardiac resynchronization therapy (CRT) is beneficial for some patients.

Generally, patients with heart failure have a poor prognosis unless the cause is correctable. Mortality rate in 1 year after the first hospitalization for HF is about 30 %. In chronic HF, mortality depends on severity of symptoms and ventricular dysfunction and can range from 10 % to 40 % a year. Specific factors that suggest a poor prognosis include hypotension, low EF, presence of CAD, troponin release, elevation of BUN, reduced GFR, hyponatremia, and poor exercise capacity.

Arterial hypertension is considered to be the most important modifiable condition in the prevention or delay of progression of heart failure. In our case the patient should be treated for arterial hypertension as a primary cause of heart failure with antihypertensive drugs and diuretics (considering that he has diastolic failure, the drug of choice should be a combination of a calcium channel blocker with hydrochlorothiazide and additional ACE-I if needed). The patient should restrict salt intake, since consuming excessive amount of sodium has been considered as one of the main triggers of the development of arterial hypertension and progression of congestive heart failure as well. At this initial stage of heart failure, the prognosis is good, and in case of patient's compliance, signs of heart failure might completely reverse. If the patient is not compliant and would not follow recommended treatment, heart failure will progress, and his condition will worsen up to the development of bilateral heart failure and generalized edema with a rather poor prognosis.

Question 11   One of the students from the group summarizes the whole case chronologically in a few minutes.

Hints for Peer Teachers

If necessary, you can help the students to summarize using the following format:

During the office hour I saw a … year old man/woman with complaints of … Patient has … as relevant prehistory. Relevant medication is…..

The major problem during history taking is … During the physical examination I saw … Additional test showed … (special findings or negative findings). In conclusion, I saw a … year old man/woman with probably … (working diagnosis) for which I want to start … (additional testing or policy). In the differential diagnosis I still consider…..

Appendix

Exemplary CBCR Case 3

A 47-Year-Old Woman with Fatigue

Consultant Version

Designed by Charles Magee, M.D., M.P.H., Mary Kwok, M.D., Jeremy Perkins, M.D. and Steven Durning, M.D., Ph.D.

Introduction

The differential diagnosis for the complaint of fatigue is exceptionally broad, encompassing nearly every organ system. A detailed history and examination supported by a careful review of systems reveal important clinical information to inform the clinician and focus the diagnostic evaluation of fatigue.

Objective

After discussing the case, students will have knowledge of different causes of fatigue and a diagnostic framework to approach patients presenting with fatigue. Students will be able to provide a differential diagnosis according to clinical history, physical examination, and basic diagnostic laboratory testing. Students will learn treatment strategies.

Preparation

Students are instructed to complete case questions in advance of the interactive session.

Background Literature for all Students

- Harrison's Principles of Internal Medicine 19th Ed, Chapters 29, 126–129
- Kochar's Clinical Medicine for Students p. 25–30; 569–598
- Robbins Basic Pathology 9th ed. p. 408–424

Additional Background Literature for Peer Teachers

- DeLoughery TG. Microcytic Anemia. NEJM. 2014;371:1324–31
- Weiss G and Goodnogh LT. Anemia of chronic disease. NEJM. 2005;352:1011–23
- Tefferi A, Hanson CA, Inwards DJ. How to Interpret and Pursue an Abnormal Complete Blood Cell Count in Adults. Mayo Clin Proc. 2005;80(7):923–936

Assessment

Students: Active participation in the session, 1 point; absent or present but not actively participating, 0 points.

Peer teachers: Excellent preparation and leadership of the session, 2 points; sufficient preparation and deficient leadership, 1 point; poor preparation and leadership, 0 points.

Proposed Time Schedule

Total 2 h (including 15 min break)
Stage 1–3   30 min
Stage 4   25 min
Stage 5   20 min
Stage 6   20 min
Short presentation 10 min

Stage 1: Presentation of the Patient's Problem
Your patient is a 47-year-old woman presenting in your outpatient clinic with increasing fatigue over the preceding month. She was previously active in yoga but has not been able to exercise due to the fatigue.

Question 1   What is your first presumption about the main problem of the patient, and what would be your first focus of history questions and physical examination?

Hints for Peer Teachers

The patient's complaint is unrefined but has several details that already allow students to begin conceptualizing the problem (i.e., duration, progression, impact). Students should first focus on conceptualizing the complaint of fatigue with a detailed history. Once the fatigue is conceptualized, a systematic approach to data collection will help narrow the broad differential.

Background Information for the Consultant

To address the adult patient experiencing fatigue, students need to conduct a careful history for key factors to conceptualize the fatigue. Inquiring of symptom onset, timing and progression, character and severity, exacerbating and alleviating factors, and associated symptoms is important to achieving this first step.

Most often, fatigue can be conceptualized into several broad categories: somnolence or sleepiness, dyspnea or shortness of breath, muscular weakness or exhaustion, psychological distress, or global neurological deficit or dysfunction. Once conceptualized, a systematic review of systems will identify organ systems spared or with potential involvement and is an important step to focus the diagnostic workup.

Handout is shown on the screen and read out loud.

> **Stage 2: Results of Initial History Taking**
> *The patient reports first noticing the fatigue when she was exerting herself and felt winded earlier than usual in yoga sessions about 6 weeks ago. She thought she may be getting out of shape and found it increasingly difficult to just keep up with her routine yoga maneuvers. Around 2 weeks ago, she noticed she was short of breath while walking during a recent shopping trip and felt her heart was beating very fast. She even notices her heart racing with light activities now, such as folding clothes. The fatigue always improves when she stops to catch her breath but gets winded when she starts up again. She's frustrated by her inability to do many of her usual activities, and her daughter noticed she was out of breath when answering the phone earlier this week. She has never experienced anything like this before and says she can't go on like this anymore.*
>
> *The patient's general medical history is notable only for G2P2 with C-section x2, with children now 19 and 22 of age. She has had no other surgeries, reports no drug allergies, and only takes a daily multivitamin when she remembers and ibuprofen. She has never used tobacco products and drinks alcohol several nights a week with dinner but has not done so in recent weeks because of her fatigue. She denies illicit substance use and is married in a monogamous relationship with her husband. Her family history is notable for her father having a myocardial infarction at age 55 and colon cancer at age 68. Her mother is alive but had a hysterectomy in her fifties. She has a single male sibling remaining, and one died in an automobile accident several years ago.*
>
> *On review of systems, she denies headaches or vision changes but notes occasionally feeling lightheaded and with graying of her vision when she to do too much; one time she noticed numbness in her fingers but that improved with rest. She denies any falls, passing out, or seizures and feels aware of her surroundings without changes in her memory or executive function. She reports getting a solid 8 h of sleep each night but doesn't feel rested in the morning. She does not feel stressed or depressed but is getting anxious about what could be causing her to feel so lousy. She denies chest pain but reports palpitations with any activity. She has not passed out though at times thought she might. She is easily winded but has no cough and is able to get a full breath of air without difficulty. She has maintained a normal appetite and continues her regular diet but does note some abdominal discomfort after meals; she reports no change in stools. She reports no dysuria, frequency, or urgency but indicates her menstrual cycles have grown erratic; she attributes this to impending menopause. She denies muscle aches or pains but feels her muscles fatigue very quickly and burn if she doesn't take a rest. She has no joint pain or swelling and reports no rashes or skin problems.*

Question 2 Based on these findings, what would be your next step of investigation?

Hints for Peer Teachers

Systematically reviewing the information, compose a prioritized problem list. Have students commit to a lead diagnosis and important diagnoses to evaluate further. With this list, identify what tests are most likely to establish or eliminate the diagnoses in consideration.

Background Information for the Consultant

The diagnostic approach to the patient with suspicion for anemia begins on initial history and physical examination and confirmation of clinical suspicion with diagnostic laboratory testing. Emphasize prioritization in the history for the pertinent positives that all align well with anemia as a cause of dyspnea and exertional intolerance rather than somnolence, psychological distress, or neurologic compromise. Make note that there may be overlap, and subtleties in history taking will help differentiate muscular exhaustion from dyspnea.

Handout is shown on the screen and read out loud.

Stage 3: Results of Diagnostic Tests

A complete blood count was performed and demonstrated hemoglobin of 8.6 g/dL and hematocrit of 25 %.

Question 3 What is now your first presumption about the main problem of the patient? Classify the hematology findings in three classes. What does this tell you about the severity? Which organ systems are possibly involved in this problem?

Hints for Peer Teachers

– Remember, anemia is a "sign" of an underlying process (similar to a fever) and should prompt a clinician into determining the etiologic cause.
– Address risk for attribution bias – attributing anemia as the principle factor for the patient's chief complaint. Does this influence possible/suspected organ system involvement?
– Make use of available classification systems – define microcytic, macrocytic, and normocytic anemia – RBC morphology, and indices vs pathophysiologic approach, as a framework to guide clinical inquiry. Explain the absolute reticulocyte count equation.
– Consider chronicity as a relevant indicator of potential pathophysiologic processes.

Background Information for the Consultant

Anemia is generally defined as a decrease in the number of circulating red blood cells and is measured by the hemoglobin or hematocrit, which provides equivalent information and is interchangeable.

Numerical definitions of anemia were first developed in 1933 based on medical student and technician values and remain the standard today. This definition lacks consideration for factors influencing hemoglobin and hematocrit other than gender, including race/ethnicity, degree of exercise/sport, and age, and up to 5 % of the general, healthy population may fall outside of the range of normal.

Reference values		
	Female	Male
Hgb (grams/dL)	12–16	14–18
Hct (%)	37–47	40–54

Initial laboratory tests include complete blood count with indices and reticulocyte count.

Classification according to qualitative and quantitative microscopic analysis is a widely accepted approach to anemia. Indices of red blood cell morphology including size (microcytic, normocytic, or macrocytic; represented by *mean corpuscular volume – MCV*), color (hypochromic, normochromic, hyperchromic; represented by *mean corpuscular hemoglobin concentration – MCHC*), shape and variation in red cell volume (*reticulocyte distribution width – RDW*), and measures of erythropoietic response (*absolute reticulocyte count – ARC*) provide an initial framework for approaching anemia. A good first step is to classify the anemia as microcytic, normocytic, or macrocytic.

Absolute reticulocyte count equation

$$\text{ARC}(\text{thousand}/\mu L) = \text{reticulocyte } \% \times \text{RBC count}(\text{million}/\mu L) \times 10$$

Example
Reticulocyte % = 2.1 %
RBC count = 3.1 million/µL
ARC (thousand/µL) = 2.1 % × 3.1 (million/µL) × 10 = 65.1 (thousand/µL)

Microcytic anemia (low MCV, <80 fL)	ARC <100,000/µL ➔ iron deficiency, anemia of chronic disease, sideroblastic anemia
	ARC >100,000/µL ➔ evaluate for hemoglobinopathy (i.e., thalassemia)
Normocytic anemia (normal MCV, 80–100 fL)	ARC <100,000/µL ➔ underproduction anemia
	ARC >100,000/µL ➔ significant recent hemorrhage or ongoing hemolysis
Macrocytic anemia (high MCV, >100 fL)	ARC <100,000/µL ➔ megaloblastic, non-megaloblastic, spurious macrocytosis
	ARC >100,000/µL ➔ evaluate for hemolysis

Question 4 What is the most likely cause of the complaints at this moment? List all possible causes of the problem and classify them in three groups: most likely, less likely, and not very likely but not excluded.

Hints for Peer Teachers

Assist the students to create a table with different conditions that can lead to anemia, and classify them in three groups, each containing at least four causes. The result should generally look like the following table (one in each category is given):

Most likely	Less likely	Not very likely
Iron deficiency	Microangiopathic hemolytic anemia (MAHA – TTP/HUS, DIC)	Marrow replacement or infiltration (primary hematopoietic malignancy, MDS, or metastatic disease)

Let the students explain/argue why they classify the conditions in the concerning groups, and let them give examples of specific diseases.

Background Information for the Consultant

Most likely	Less likely	Not very likely
Iron deficiency	Microangiopathic hemolytic anemia (MAHA – TTP/HUS, DIC)	Marrow replacement or infiltration (primary hematopoietic malignancy, MDS, multiple myeloma, or metastatic disease)
B12 deficiency	Systemic lupus erythematosus (SLE)	Mechanical trauma
Folate deficiency	Glucose-6-phosphate dehydrogenase deficiency (G6PD)	Malaria infection
Hypothyroidism	Sickle cell anemia	Thalassemia
Anemia of chronic disease/inflammation	Thalassemia	Paroxysmal nocturnal hemoglobinuria
Chronic/subacute blood loss (gastrointestinal, gynecologic, blood donor)		Aplastic anemia

Appendix 171

Question 5 Agree upon the most relevant hypotheses, and discuss their cause or pathology on organ level or on a more detailed level. Is there a problem in anatomical, cellular, or biochemical respect?

Hints for Peer Teachers

Undifferentiated anemia requires clinical categorization according to (1) underproduction, (2) destruction/hemolysis, or (3) blood loss:

- Underproduction anemias result from loss of stimulus related to disruption of cell signaling and nutritional deficiencies in reticulocyte cytoplasmic or nucleic synthetic processes.
- Hemolysis is associated with structural and physiologic limitations, in addition to immune, trauma-, or infection-mediated destruction.
- Anemia from blood loss can result from acute, subacute, or chronic loss due to organ-specific pathology; most commonly implicated organs include menorrhagia and gastrointestinal blood loss (must rule out malignancy).

Guide the group in elaborating the three types of anemia by using the three charts below for your reference

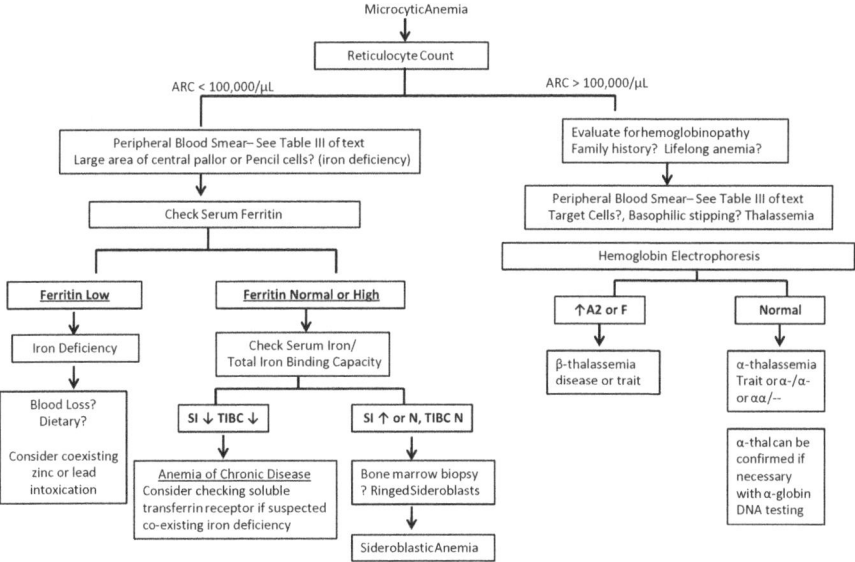

Appendix

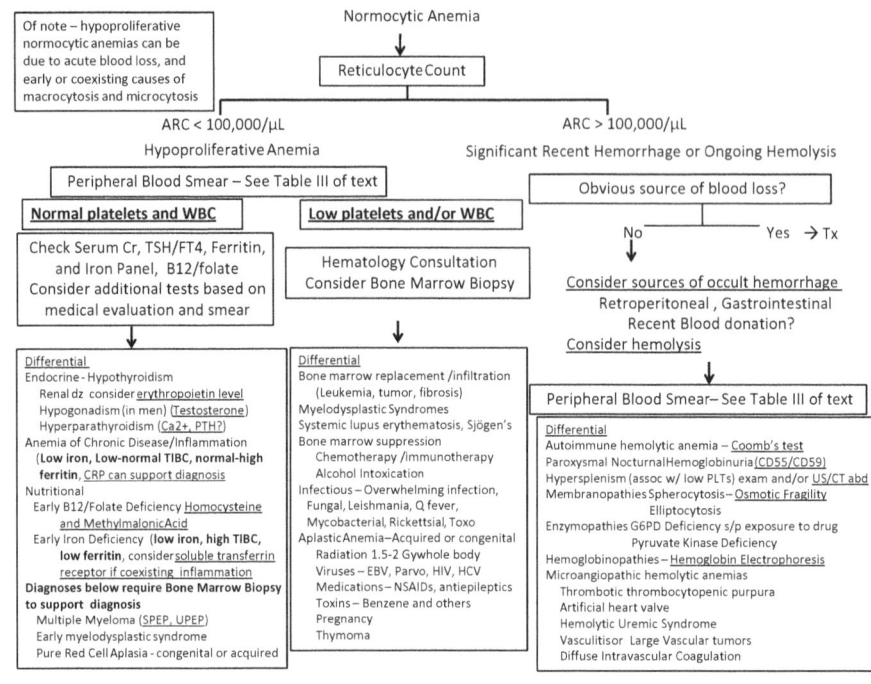

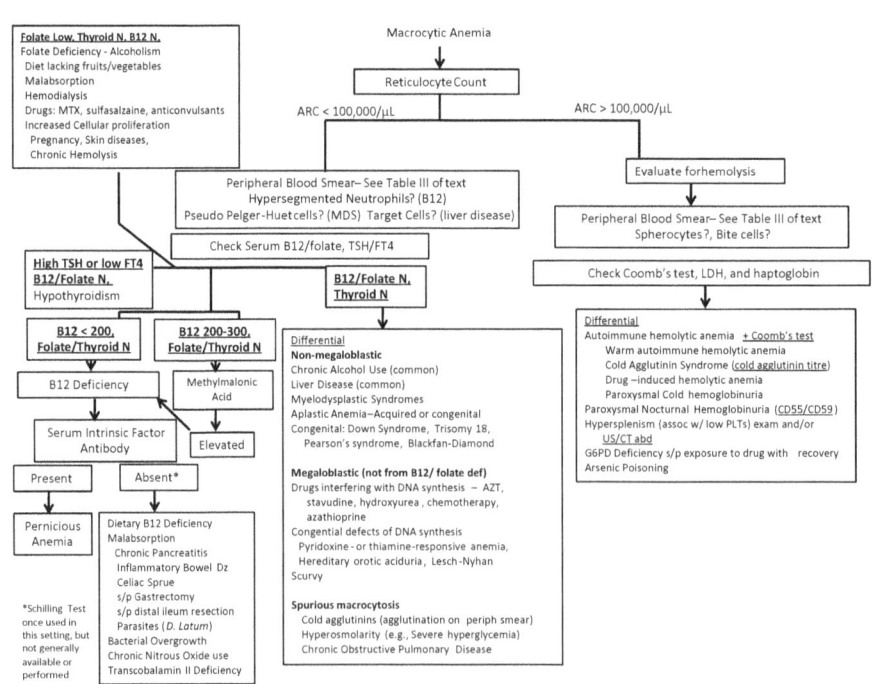

Appendix

Background Information for the Consultant

Microcytic Anemia

Categorization according to absolute reticulocyte count provides insight into proliferative status. ARC <100,000/μL indicates iron deficiency, anemia of chronic disease/inflammation, or sideroblastic anemia. ARC >100,000/μL points to a hemoglobinopathy such as thalassemia.

- The most common hypoproliferative, microcytic anemia is iron-deficiency anemia, accounting for up to 50 % of anemia worldwide:
  - Classically described as a microcytic, hypochromic anemia.
  - May have a concomitant reactive thrombocytosis.
  - Peripheral blood smear may demonstrate anisocytosis, poikilocytosis, and elliptocytosis.
  - Diagnostic studies for iron deficiency include serum iron and total iron-binding capacity (TIBC), serum ferritin, and transferrin saturation.
  - Low ferritin is diagnostic of iron deficiency; however ferritin can be elevated in inflammatory states, so normal or elevated ferritin does not rule out iron deficiency and can mask negative iron balance.
  - Iron-deficient states occur due to (1) increased demand for iron, (2) increased loss of iron, and (3) decreased intake or absorption.
  - Chronic blood loss (chronic iron consumption) as seen with menstrual irregularity diagnoses leads to iron deficiency, as well as pregnancy in nutritionally deficient regions worldwide.
  - Additional nutritional deficiencies can present concomitantly and potentially mask iron deficiency or the additional deficiency(ies) according to mean corpuscular volume; reticulocyte distribution width (RDW) helps distinguish these entities.

Iron nutritional states and anemia					
	Normal	Negative iron balance	Iron-deficient erythropoiesis	Early iron-deficient anemia	Late iron-deficiency anemia
RBC morphology	Normal	Normal	Normal	Mild hypochromia, anisocytosis, poikilocytosis	Mod-severe hypochromia, anisocytosis, poikilocytosis with target, and pencil-shaped cells
RBC indices (MCV, RDW)	Normal	Normal	MCV normal, RDW ↑	MCV ↓ RDW ↑	MCV ↓↓ RDW normal
Ferritin	Normal	↓	↓	↓↓	↓↓
Transferrin saturation	Normal	Normal	↓	↓↓	↓↓
TIBC	Normal	↑	↑	↑	↑

RBC red blood cell, *MCV* mean corpuscular volume, *RDW* reticulocyte distribution width, *TIBC* total iron-binding capacity, ↓ reduced, ↓↓ markedly reduced, ↑ elevated, ↑↑ markedly elevated

- Anemia of chronic disease/inflammation is important to differentiate from iron deficiency and reflects impaired provision of iron to marrow for sufficient hemoglobin synthesis, inflammatory cytokine inhibition of erythropoietin production, and stimulation of marrow RBC production:
  - Normal/elevated ferritin in setting of reduced serum iron, transferrin saturation, and microcytic, hypochromic RBC morphology is supportive of anemia of chronic disease/inflammation over iron-deficiency anemia.
  - Concomitant iron deficiency can be treated and will generally restore iron stores; however, it will not correct anemia of chronic disease/inflammation.
  - The soluble transferrin receptor can be used to distinguish between iron deficiency (increased) and anemia of chronic disease (normal) and will be increased when both processes are present.
- Thalassemia is a hemoglobinopathy typically presenting as a microcytic, normoproductive anemia due to defective globin chain synthesis; peripheral blood smears typically demonstrate target cells. Hemoglobin electrophoresis is a cost-effective screening tool when clinically suspected.
- Endocrinopathies implicated in microcytic anemia include hyperparathyroidism and male hypogonadism (low testosterone).
- Bicytopenia or pancytopenia (low white blood cell count, platelets, or both) may suggest either bone marrow failure or bone marrow infiltrative process; bone marrow biopsy may be indicated.
- Sideroblastic anemia is uncommon. It is often micro- or normocytic and characterized by normal iron indices but impaired utilization of iron into hemoglobin.

Diagnostic considerations in microcytic anemia					
Differential tests	Iron deficiency	[Chronic] inflammation	Renal disease[a]	Thalassemia	Sideroblastic anemia
Degree of anemia	Mild-severe	Mild	Mild-severe	Mild-severe	Moderate-severe
MCV (fL)	60–90	80–90	90	<80	Low-normal (inherited); high (acquired)
Morphology	Normo-microcytic	Normo-microcytic	Normocytic	Microcytic	Variable
Serum iron	<30	<50	Normal	Normal-high	Normal-high
TIBC	>360	<300	Normal	Normal	Normal
Iron saturation (%)	<10	10–20	Normal	Normal (30–80)	Normal (30–80)
Serum ferritin (g/dL)	<15	30–200	115–150	50–300	50–300
Iron stores	0	2–4+	1–4+	Elevated	Normal
Hgb electrophoresis	Normal	Normal	Normal	Abnormal (β-thalassemia; α-thalassemia can be normal)	Normal

Adapted from Harrisons Principles of Internal Medicine, 18th Ed, Chapter 103, Tables 103-4 and 103-6

MCV mean corpuscular volume, *TIBC* total iron-binding capacity, *Hgb* hemoglobin

[a]Anemia from "Renal Disease" may have similar characteristics with anemia from [chronic] inflammation

Normocytic Anemia

Categorization according to ARC provides insight into proliferative status

- Hypoproliferative anemia is characterized by ARC <100,000/μL and can occur with:
  - Acute blood loss (pre-hemodilution) or with early or coexisting micro- and macrocytic anemia
  - Acute autoimmune processes (such as SLE flare, Sjögren's syndrome flare)
  - Acute infections (including fungal, leishmania, Q fever, rickettsia, mycobacteria, toxoplasmosis, or overwhelming bacterial infection)
  - Infiltrative marrow process such as multiple myeloma
  - Marrow suppressive conditions including post-chemotherapy or immunotherapy
  - Anemia of chronic disease/inflammation
- Aplastic anemia is either congenital or acquired and typically manifests as pancytopenia; acquired may result from whole-body radiation (>1.5 Gy), viral infection (EBV, parvo-B19, HIV, HCV), medications (NSAIDs, antiepileptics), benzene exposure, thymoma, or even pregnancy. Pure red cell aplasia may present as isolated anemia and is associated with parvo-B19 infection.
- ARC >100,000/μL indicates significant recent hemorrhage or broadly encompasses active hemolytic processes. An unremarkable search for obvious blood loss may be reasonably followed with evaluation for occult blood loss and hemolytic process.
  - Hemolytic anemia is generally classified into the following categories:

Intrinsic, inherited:

- Enzyme deficiency, such as X-linked G6PD deficiency, whereby erythrocytes are unable to compensate for specific oxidative stressors (infections, medications including primaquine, sulfonamides, nitrofurantoin, and vitamin K derivatives) through impaired regeneration of GSH. Peripheral blood smear may demonstrate spherocytes or bite cells.
- Hemoglobinopathies – Sickle cell anemia remains the prototype, brought about by deoxygenated hemoglobin S distortion into long polymers that become irreversibly sickled; thalassemias are discussed in microcytic anemia.
- Hereditary spherocytosis, an autosomal dominant inherited disorder of nondeformable spherocyte morphology that is unable to pass through splenic cords and remains sequestered in the spleen; splenectomy corrects the anemia,

Intrinsic, acquired:

- Paroxysmal nocturnal hemoglobinuria, resulting from an acquired somatic mutation of the PIGA gene, results in erythrocytes exceptionally vulnerable to complement-mediated lysis; therapies to block the terminal complement membrane attack complex reduce hemolysis yet expose patients to encapsulated bacterial infections.

Extrinsic

- Immune-mediated, includes a range of antibody-mediated erythrocyte destruction, including warm antibody (idiopathic, CLL, SLE, drug-mediated), cold antibody (idiopathic, infectious mononucleosis/EBV, mycoplasma infection, B cell neoplasms)
- Mechanical shearing with artificial heart valves or repetitive tissue trauma (runner's anemia or march hemoglobinuria).
- Microangiopathic hemolytic anemia (MAHA) and/or disseminated intravascular coagulation (DIC) whereby RBC trauma occurs in small vessels with disrupted luminal surface. Peripheral smear reveals schistocytes in TTP, HUS, aHUS, and other thrombotic microangiopathies.
- Direct infections and toxins, such as with erythrocytic parasites including malaria and babesiosis

Macrocytic Anemia

Categorization according to ARC provides insight into proliferative status.

- ARC <100,000/μL indicates hypoproliferative state. Megaloblastic anemias manifest due to impaired DNA synthesis and include vitamin B12 and folate deficiency. As the name implies, neutrophil "hypersegmentation" (more than 5), macro-ovalocytes, poikilocytosis, and anisocytosis are common peripheral blood smear findings.
    - Vitamin B12 deficiency can result from nutritional scarcity (vegetarian) as well as pernicious anemia, an autoimmune attack on gastric parietal cells elaborating intrinsic factor for gastrointestinal absorption of vitamin B12. Celiac disease, IBD, chronic pancreatitis, and gastrectomy can also impact dietary absorption, as can bacterial overgrowth and, in the developing world, fish tapeworms. Replete stores are sufficient for approximately 2–3 years.
    - Folate is present in leafy green vegetables, and deficiency can arise in 2 or 3 months, commonly seen with alcoholism, impaired gastrointestinal absorption, metabolic interference from medications (methotrexate, pyrimethamine, trimethoprim), or increased demand (chronic anemia, pregnancy, malignancy, hemodialysis).

Appendix 177

- Non-megaloblastic, hypoproliferative, macrocytic anemias are associated with liver disease, alcoholism (via marrow suppression), myelodysplastic syndrome, hypothyroidism (as well as hypoproliferative microcytic anemia), or medications that directly limit DNA synthesis, such as chemotherapeutics.

Question 6 Which questions must be asked to discriminate between the most relevant hypotheses?

Hints for Peer Teachers

It is important that students thoroughly create questions and know why they need to be asked. Questions should be formulated so that they either confirm or reject a hypothetical diagnosis.

Background Information for the Consultant

The questions that can be asked are:

- Dietary history, change in diet
- Fever, recent or current infections
- Abdominal pain
- Nausea and vomiting (hematemesis)
- Cough and hemoptysis
- Anorexia
- Urine coloration (hematuria)
- Jet-black, dark maroon, or bright-red stools (melenic stool, hematochezia)
- "Pica," crunching ice, eating clay, chalk, laundry starch
- Dizziness, tiredness, easy fatigability
- Rashes or easy bruising
- Use of medications, current and recent
- Use of alcohol, current and recent
- History of cancer, "B" symptoms
- Menstrual and pregnancy history
- History of mechanical heart valve/left ventricular assist device – LVAD
- Family history of anemia
- Exposure history, including heavy metals, lead, benzene, radiation, chemotherapy

Handout is shown on the screen and read out loud.

> **Stage 4: Results of Additional Focused History**
> The patient states she eats a balanced vegetarian diet and reports she has had increasing abdominal discomfort in recent weeks following meals. She denies any recent infections and has not noticed any gross bleeding associated with cough, vomiting, defecation, or urination. She has observed no rashes and reports soft, brown stools once daily though has had occasional dark stools in recent weeks. Her menses have recently become erratic, occasionally quite heavy and variable ranging from 1 to 4 weeks apart and lasting for several weeks each time for several months. She reports using ibuprofen 800 mg up to three times a day as needed for knee pain with physical activity and menstrual cramping as needed, as well as a daily multivitamin. She is unaware of any possible exposure to lead or radiation. She reports no personal history of cancer, and review of systems is negative for fevers, chills, weight loss, or night sweats. She is unaware if other family members have anemia or other active health issues.

Question 7 How does the history of the patient influence your differential diagnosis? First think of only the three big categories of causes.

Hints for Peer Teachers

Use the following table for the history information to differentiate between the most likely hypotheses. Add a plus (+) in the table if the history question is likely to be answered affirmative and a minus (−) if the answer of the history question is likely to be answered negative. Add a plus/minus (+/−) if both are applicable or if they do not differentiate enough.

History information	Decreased production	Increased destruction	Blood loss
Dietary history, change in diet	+	+/−	+/−
Etc.			

Background Information for the Consultant

They can be written in the table as below

History information	Decreased production	Increased destruction	Blood loss
Dietary history, change in diet	+	+/−	+/−
Fever, recent or current infections	+	+	+/−
Abdominal pain	−	+	+

(continued)

History information	Decreased production	Increased destruction	Blood loss
Nausea and vomiting (hematemesis)	+	−	+
Cough and hemoptysis	−	−	+
Anorexia	+/−	−	+
Urine coloration (hematuria)	−	+	−/+
Jet-black, dark, maroon, or bright-red stools (melena, hematochezia)	+/−	−	+
Pale-colored stools	−	+	−
"Pica," crunching ice, eating clay, chalk, laundry starch	+	−	−/+
Dizziness, tiredness, easy fatigability	+	+	+
Rashes or easy bruising	−	+	−/+
Use of medications, current and recent	+/− (specifics)	+/− (specifics)	+/− (specifics)
Use of alcohol, current and recent	+	−	+
History of cancer, "B" symptoms	+	−	−
Menstrual and pregnancy history	+	−	+
History of mechanical heart valve/left ventricular assist device – LVAD	−	+	−
Family history of anemia	+	+/−	
Exposure history, including heavy metals, lead, benzene, radiation, chemotherapy	+	−/+	−

Question 8 **Which parts of the physical examination are required in order to exclude some unlikely but important hypotheses?**

Hints for Peer Teachers

Let the students suggest specific physical examination maneuvers they want to perform. Ask them what they expect from the findings of the examinations and how each maneuver will influence the differential diagnosis.

Make with the group a table of all unlikely but important causes, and list what the group would expect to find with physical examination related to these diseases using + and −.

Background Information for the Consultant

Unlikely but important hypotheses					
Findings with Px	Gastrointestinal bleeding	Disseminated intravascular coagulopathy	Aplastic anemia	Thalassemia	Malaria
Melena	+	−	−	−	−
Hemoptysis	+/−	−	−	−	−
Petechiae	−	+	−	−	+/− (rare)
Purpura	−	+	+/−	−	+/−

(continued)

Findings with Px	Gastrointestinal bleeding	Disseminated intravascular coagulopathy	Aplastic anemia	Thalassemia	Malaria
Ecchymoses	−	+	+	−	−
Conjunctival pallor	+	+	+	+/−	+
Fever	−	+/−	−	−	+
Splenomegaly	−	+/− (rare)	+	+	+

Unlikely but important hypotheses (section header above table)

Handout is shown on the screen and read out loud

Stage 5: Results of a Focused Physical Examination

On examination, the general condition of the patient was not ill. Her temperature was 37.0 °C. She had a blood pressure of 119/68 mmHg with a heart rate of 106 bpm. The color of the skin was pale with subconjunctival pallor. Further examination of the skin did not reveal petechiae, purpura, or ecchymoses. Capillary refill was delayed to 3 s and conjunctival pallor evident. Cardiac auscultation revealed a normal S1 and S2 and a two out of six systolic ejection murmur. Jugular venous distension measured approximately 6 cm. Chest excursion is equal and symmetric, and on auscultation, normal breath sounds are heard without wheeze, rub, or rhonchus. On abdominal examination, there was mild tenderness to epigastric palpation only and no hepatosplenomegaly. On auscultation there were normal peristaltic sounds; ascites was not present and palpable lymph nodes were not enlarged. Rectal vault was empty w/o no visible blood. Extremities are notable for no edema or lesions and intact pulses.

Question 9 Which hypotheses now remain in the differential diagnosis to be investigated further?

Hints for Peer Teachers

Use the following table for the physical examination findings. Add a plus (+) in the table if the fining is likely to be answered affirmative and a minus (−) if the answer of the finding is likely to be answered negative. Add a plus/minus (+/−) if both are applicable or if they do not differentiate. What diagnoses has become more likely now?

Appendix

Physical examination findings	Decreased production	Increased destruction	Blood loss
VS – HR 106			
Skin – pale; subconjunctival pallor			
Delayed capillary refill			
No petechiae, purpura, or ecchymoses			
2/6 systolic murmur			
6 cm JVD			
Epigastric pain			
No splenomegaly			
No hepatomegaly			

Background Information for the Consultant

The purpose of the physical examination is to assess the severity and possible causes of jaundice. Findings can be added to the table as shown below

Physical examination findings	Decreased production	Increased destruction	Blood loss
VS – HR 106	+	+	+
Skin – pale; subconjunctival pallor	+	+	+
Delayed capillary refill	+	+	+
No petechiae, purpura, or ecchymoses	+/−	−	+/−
2/6 systolic murmur	+	+	+
6 cm JVD	+	−	+/−
Epigastric pain	−	+	−
No splenomegaly	+/−	−	+/−
No hepatomegaly	−	−	−

Based on the nonspecific findings on the physical examination (tachycardia, pale skin, delayed capillary refill, subconjunctival pallor), combined with the absence of splenomegaly, petechiae, purpura, or ecchymoses, evidence of overt or occult blood loss makes focusing the differential diagnosis difficult. In fact, the physical examination may be inappropriately reassuring in mildly anemic patients.

Question 10   Which diagnostic investigations need to be done to confirm or exclude remaining diagnoses?

Hints for Peer Teachers

List all the diagnostic procedures that are thought to be essential. Consider the diagnostic value and cost of the tests (cost-effectiveness).

Let students think about laboratory and supplementary investigations (e.g., full blood count, reticulocyte count, hemoglobin electrophoresis, etc.), which can enable them to formulate diagnosis.

Background Information for the Consultant

The following initial investigations are recommended:

- Full blood count: Hgb, MCV, RDW
- Reticulocyte count, ARC
- Peripheral blood smear
- Iron panel: serum iron, TIBC; ferritin; transferrin saturation
- B12/folate panel: B12, folate, methylmalonic acid, homocysteine
- Haptoglobin
- Direct antiglobulin test (DAT, aka Coombs test)
- Complete metabolic profile (basic metabolic profile and liver function tests)

Additional tests to consider to investigate specific diagnoses:

- Urinalysis: microscopic hematuria (RBCs), proteinuria, bilirubin, urobilinogen
- Coagulation panel: PT, PTT, INR
- Stool guaiac test
- G6PD level (activity)
- Hemoglobin electrophoresis
- Osmotic fragility test
- Bone marrow biopsy
- Rapid malaria test
- Monospot (heterophile Ab test)
- EBV IgM, IgG
- ANA, anti-dsDNA, anti-Sm, or antiphospholipid Abs
- Flow cytometry (CD55, CD59)
- Erythropoietin level

Handout is shown on the screen and read out loud.

Stage 6: Results of Diagnostic Tests
Full blood count:

- *RBC count – 3.4 million (normal range in adult woman: 4.2–5.4 million cells/mm^3)*
- *Hgb – 8.6 gm/dL (normal range in adult woman: 12–16 gm/dL)*
- *Hct – 25 % (normal range in adult woman: 37–47 %)*
- *MCV – 73 fL (85–98 fL)*
- *RDW – 18 % (11.5–14.5 %)*

Reticulocyte count:

- *1.1 %*

(continued)

Peripheral blood smear

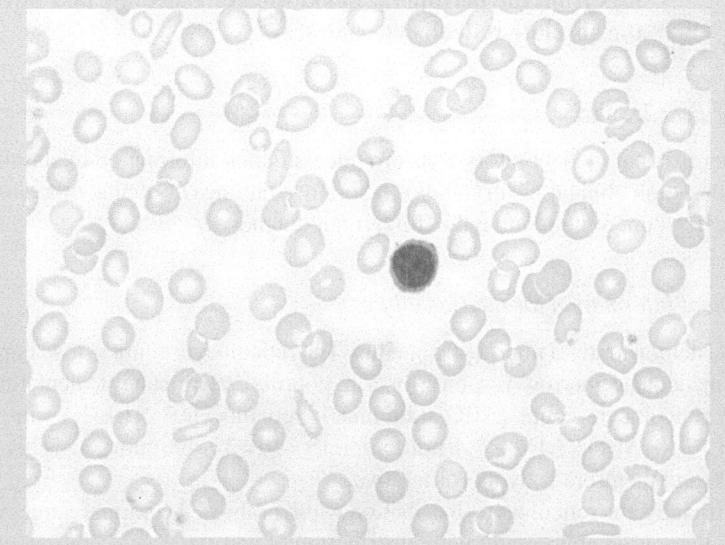

Peripheral blood smear, 40×: hypochromia, microcytosis with mild poikilocytosis, including target and pencil-shaped cells.

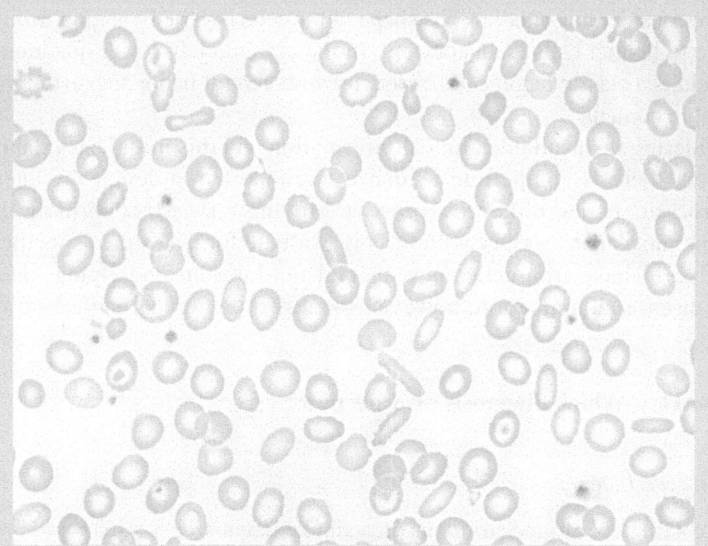

Peripheral blood smear, 40×: hypochromia, microcytosis with anisocytosis and poikilocytosis, including target and pencil-shaped cells.

Question 11 Interpret the findings from the diagnostic tests. How much certainty do they give about the hypotheses? What are the key findings from the peripheral blood smear? Calculate and interpret the absolute reticulocyte count.

Hints for Peer Teachers

Do these results of the laboratory tests provide sufficient information to classify the anemia based on clinical history and/or laboratory findings? Calculate the absolute reticulocyte count to help refine the differential diagnosis.

Background Information for the Consultant

The CBC demonstrates a microcytic anemia. The reticulocyte count is low, concerning for inadequate marrow response or a hypoproliferative state. Calculating the absolute reticulocyte count (ARC thou/mm^3) = reticulocyte % × RBC count (million/mm^3) × 10; ARC = 1.1% × 3.4(million/mm^3) × 10 = 37,400/mm^3. This is <100,000 and therefore is hypoproliferative.

Additionally, the reticulocyte distribution width is above the normal range, which suggests there is an abnormally wide distribution of cell sizes, as is consistent with a mixed population in an evolving nutritionally deficient state.

Lastly, the peripheral smear provides valuable morphologic information. The visualized RBCs appear small as compared to the lymphocyte that might be used for reference in the field (expect 1.5× size of mature RBC); in this case, some of the RBCs are considerably smaller. The shape of the cells is varied, ranging from biconcave disc to helmet cells (schistocytes). In the extreme left, lower quadrant of the visual field is a classic target cell (codocyte) with central pallor suggesting reduced hemoglobin content.

Considering the available clinical information and this initial basic laboratory evaluation, there is compelling evidence to support iron-deficiency anemia as the microcytic, hypoproliferative process. Moving forward, confirming the suspected diagnosis is necessary with tests to evaluate for iron stores specifically. It is possible to have iron-deficiency anemia masking an underlying anemia of chronic disease/inflammation; however, there is little clinical indication for this concern.

Question 11 Which diagnosis prevails now?

Hints for Peer Teachers

Are there sufficient grounds to focus on a single diagnosis?

Appendix

Background Information for the Consultant

The most likely diagnosis for this patient is iron-deficiency anemia. Applied to this clinical case, this patient may have peptic ulcer disease relating to the chronic, high-dose NSAID usage or *Helicobacter pylori*, or otherwise relating to the irregular menses, best characterized in this case as metromenorrhagia. Diagnosing iron deficiency requires investigation for the etiology, whether nutritionally deficient diet or significant blood loss exceeding physiologic stores and compensatory mechanisms.

As the most common cause of anemia worldwide, the etiology is varied. In the USA, chronic blood loss is the most common etiology, as is suggested by the case presented here. In the developing world, nutritional deficiencies are more common and complicated by the presence of parasitic infections competing for precious dietary iron with the host, particularly in children and women of childbearing age.

To confirm the diagnosis, serum iron, TIBC, ferritin, and transferrin saturation are indicated laboratory studies. In addition to confirming iron deficiency, these laboratory studies may shed light on the presence of a concomitant anemia of chronic disease/inflammation if present (though not clinically supported in this case). To identify specific causes, consider stool guaiac and upper endoscopy to identify peptic ulcer disease and risk for Helicobacter pylori infection (recently identified as an independent cause of iron-deficiency anemia).

Question 12   Given this diagnosis and patient circumstances, which therapy or policy for care is now indicated? What is the prognosis if the patient is treated? What if the patient would not be treated?

Hints for Peer Teachers

What is the overarching treatment strategy for this condition?

Background Information for the Consultant

Identifying the underlying etiology of the iron-deficient state is paramount, as effective treatment needs to address this process; otherwise the ability to effectively treat is contingent on the severity of the underlying disease and the erythropoietic potential or regenerative capacity (generally thought to be 6–8× normal physiologic repletion).

In this case, there are two potential sources of blood loss – GI blood loss through possible peptic ulcer or *Helicobacter pylori* infection (or both) vs potential erratic and heavy menstrual cycles.

Simultaneously working to regulate menstrual irregularities and investigating for GI blood loss or *H. pylori* infection are recommended, all the while starting dietary iron supplementation.

Presentation 1   A short presentation etiology (max 10 min) is given by one of the peer teachers.

Hints for Peer Teachers

Peer teachers are asked in advance to prepare a short presentation on causes of microcytic, hypoproliferative anemias, as the most commonly encountered form of anemia.

Give a very short overview of the pathophysiology, epidemiology, symptoms, diagnostic findings, and treatment of each disease entity. Please keep it brief, especially the causes and diagnostic tests for viral hepatitis.

The mini lecture is meant to provide the students with information they can directly apply in the continuation of the case. Peer teachers should therefore make sure that the information in the mini lecture is directly applicable (i.e., explanation about pathophysiology or pros and cons of certain diagnostics). The goal of the mini lecture is not to have peer teachers comprehensively review a large topic. The purpose is not that of an examination to investigate how much this student knows; rather the mini lecture should provide all students with helpful background information to stimulate their understanding of the case: this is true peer teaching. Peer teachers should be selective in what they present, as the presentation should never take longer than 10 min and usually much shorter.

Background Information for the Consultant

The mini lecture is meant to provide the students with information they can directly apply in the continuation of the case.

The background information may be more extensive than what the peer teachers are going to tell.

Iron-Deficiency Anemia

Etiology – Iron-deficiency anemia is caused by either malabsorption of iron, deficiency of transferrin, or loss of iron.

Development – Iron deficiency develops in a series of *stages:*

Normal: storage iron repletion – ferritin normal, bone marrow iron normal, producing RBCs with normal morphology indices

Stage 1: negative iron balance/storage iron depletion – decreased ferritin with preserved transferrin saturation, increased TIBC, normal RBC morphology indices

Stage 2: early iron-deficiency/iron-deficient erythropoiesis – decreased ferritin and transferrin saturation, RBC morphology changes evident: reduced MCV, MCHC; widened RDW RBC iron is decreased **but no anemia:**

(a) TIBC increases.
(b) Serum iron decreases.
(c) Microcytic RBC develops.
(d) Hypochromic RBC develops.

Stage 3: iron-deficient anemia – all above features but with hemoglobin decrease.
Clinical signs/symptoms

Numbers

Protein	Tissue/cells	Iron, mg	Total body iron, %	Function of iron-containing structure
Hemoglobin	Red blood cells	2,500	66	To transport by blood
Myoglobin (and other nonenzyme muscle proteins)	Muscle	500	13	Transport in muscle
Heme enzymes (e.g., cytochromes, oxidoreductases)	All cells	50	1	Transport, utilization, and consumption in all cells
Nonheme iron proteins	All cells	200	~5	Transport, iron reserves in all cells
Ferritin and hemosiderin	Liver, spleen, bone marrow	500	13	Iron storage
Transferrin	Plasma and extravascular fluids	14	>1	Iron transport
Total		3,800	98	

1. Daily iron losses 1 mg/day.
2. Dietary iron is present in two forms – inorganic iron and heme iron.
3. Heme iron absorption up to 35 %, inorganic iron absorption 10 %.
4. Dietary sources of iron:

    (a) Rich sources: liver, oysters, legumes
    (b) Fair sources: beef, lamb, pork, poultry, fish
    (c) Poor sources: iron-fortified flours/cereals
    (d) Negligible sources: fruits, dairy products, spinach, raisins

5. Iron content of blood 0.5 mg/mL.
6. Normal menstrual losses 35–40 ml (17.5–20 mg).
7. Pregnancy requirements ~1,000 mg.

    Losses: 350 mg to fetus and placenta, 250 mg during delivery (500 mL blood)
    Physiologic: 240 mg for daily losses, 450 mg for increased maternal RBC mass
    Iron-Deficiency Symptoms and Signs

1. Most symptoms are secondary to the anemia and not specific to iron deficiency
2. Nonheme tissue iron loss

    (a) Headache
    (b) Tongue burning
    (c) Pica (clay, chalk), pagophagia (ice) **(specific, not sensitive)**
    (d) Nocturnal leg cramping (restless legs)

3. Signs

    (a) Glossitis (rapid turnover of epithelial cells)
    (b) Stomatitis
    (c) Angular cheilitis

4. Morphology

Peripheral blood smear reveals red blood cells are smaller (microcytic) and paler (hypochromatic). The central area of pallor which occupies approximately one third of the normal red blood cell diameter becomes much larger, and the cells have a wider distribution of size as is indicated by the increased RDW (red cell distribution width); "target cell," or codocytes on peripheral blood smear. As iron deficiency worsens, RBCs become progressively irregular in shape, with fragments and bizarre RBC forms seen with profound iron deficiency; schistocytes are seen on peripheral blood smear. Bone marrow biopsy in a patient with iron deficiency anemia shows an increase of erythroid progenitor cells and a decrease/absence of stainable iron in macrophages.

Handout is shown on the screen and read out loud.

> **Stage 7: Final Decursus**
> *The patient was diagnosed with iron-deficiency anemia. Stool guaiac was negative, and stopping NSAIDs and empiric proton-pump inhibitor therapy alleviated epigastric pain. Low-dose estrogen therapy provided regularity to menstrual cycles and reduced heaviness of flow. She started on oral iron sulfate, 325 mg three times daily for 3 months. On follow-up, Hgb increased to 11.2 gm/dL. Iron therapy was continued at twice daily for an additional 6 months at which time Hgb was 13.1 gm/dL. Education was provided to continue with dietary choices for iron-rich foods, including leafy green vegetables.*

Question 13 One of the students from the group summarizes the whole case chronologically in a few minutes, with emphasis on symptoms, physical examination, and lab tests that were critical in making the diagnosis.

Appendix

Exemplary CBCR Case 4

Two Patients with Hearing Loss

Consultant Version

Designed and revised by several authors across many years at University Medical Center Utrecht. Translated and adapted for this volume by Maria van Loon MD.

Introduction

Hearing loss is a very common complaint in all age groups, which can have major consequences. It can have a significant influence on the quality of life. Reduction of hearing may be regarded a result of a change in the function of the auditory organ. This change may occur in the ordinary course of a life process (such as wear) or may be a result of pathological disorders. The general practitioner can play an important role in the further diagnosis of hearing impairment as illustrated in this lesson.

Objective of This CBCR Case

After discussion of this case, the student can identify the many causes of hearing loss. The student can indicate what types of impairment exist and how the doctor can differentiate between the various disorders based on history and physical examination. Moreover, the student can discuss treatment options.

Preparation[4]

All students should prepare questions 1–3 of case A and questions 8 and 9 of case B at home by using the given literature.

Background literature for students

- De Jongh et al. Diagnostiek van alledaagse klachten hoofdstuk Slechter horen p. 201
- De Jongh et al. Diagnostiek van alledaagse klachten hoofdstuk Oorpijn p. 275
- NHG-standaarden "Slechthorendheid" en "Otitis media acuta"

Additional Background Literature for Peer Teachers

- Huizing et al. Leerboek keel-, neus- oorheelkunde en hoofd-halschirurgie. Hoofdstuk 2 (onderzoek oor en gehoor), hoofdstuk 3 (aandoeningen uitwendige oor), hoofdstuk 4 (aandoeningen trommelvlies en middenoor), hoofdstuk 5 (aandoeningen binnenoor)

---

[4] Preparation and assessment rules as used at UMC Utrecht – to be adapted to local requirements

Assessment

Students: Active participation in the session, 1 point; absent or present but not actively participating, 0 points.

Peer teachers: Excellent preparation and leadership of the session, 2 points; sufficient preparation and deficient leadership, 1 point; poor preparation and leadership, 0 points.

Proposed Time Schedule

Case A (question 1 t/m 7)	50 min
Mini lecture	10 min
Case B (question 8 t/m 10)	40 min
Question 11	5 min

Case A: A 63-Year-Old Lady With Hearing Loss

Stage 1: Presentation of the Patient's Problem
At your consultation you see Mrs. Mohammed. She is 63 years old, is married, and has five children. She is from Morocco but has lived for 10 years in the Netherlands. She still thinks the Dutch language is quite difficult, although she understands it reasonably if she concentrates well. Speaking is reasonable, but she still prefers to talk in her native language. You have seen her twice: once for an introductory meeting and about 2 years ago regarding to fatigue where ultimately no cause was found. Mrs. Mohammed tells you she worries about her hearing. She noticed herself that she understands people less and less, but now also her environment started to complain about her frequent "pardon/excuse me/sorry?", when she is asked or told anything.

Question 1 Identify the request for help. Why is good hearing especially important for this patient?

Background Information for the Consultant

For this "request for help," the patient's concern about her hearing loss plays a major role. It is important that students realize that hearing loss among immigrant patients can exacerbate a potential language barrier. If you cannot properly understand a conversation, speaking becomes increasingly difficult as well.

Appendix

Question 2 Make an initial classification of possible causes of the main complaint. Think about the anatomy and categories of illness first. You don't have to make a diagnosis yet.

Hints for Peer Teachers

Create a table of different groups of conditions that can lead to hearing loss. Fill the table as in the example. Think of a classification by anatomy.

Tip: Draw a blank table for the start of the lesson on the board. This saves time when you discuss the case.

Condition	History		Physical examination		Additional investigations	
	Pro	Against	Pro	Against	Pro	Against
External ear						
Middle ear						
Etc.						

Background Information for the Consultant

It is important that students end with a clear table of groups of conditions. Based on these groups, questions for history taking can be formulated later. Let the students spend relatively much time to fill in the table (about 15 min). If the table is filled in properly, discussion of the rest of the case will become clearer and therefore faster.

This is a useful classification of anatomy below (see also the table in the Appendix):

1. External ear
2. Middle ear
3. Internal ear/cochlear
4. Retro-cochlear

Examples of diagnoses can be categorized in these groups.

Question 3 What additional history questions can you think of to distinguish between the different groups of conditions?

Hints for Peer Teachers

It is important that students systematically create and use questions. Think of questions which make diagnoses listed in the previous question more or less likely. Allow the students to reason each question: why would they ask this question and, how can an answer to the question influence the differential diagnosis?

Background Information for the Consultant

Students must now consider what questions can help them in making a differential diagnosis. Even more than asking a "good question," it is important that the question helps to differentiate between the diseases.

Questions that can be used are:

- Duration and course; acute, progressive, paroxysmal (Meniere), during pregnancy/menopause (otosclerosis).
- Severity (impact on daily life).
- Uni- or bilateral (unilaterally may occur in unilateral otitis media, noise trauma, acute idiopathic hearing loss, acoustic neuroma). In otitis media and noise trauma, bilateral hearing loss is seen more often.
- Ear pain, itching, or otorrhea (otitis).
- A cold or upper respiratory infection (otitis).
- Use of antibiotics and other ototoxic drugs.
- Dizziness and tinnitus (Meniere).
- Trauma capitis.
- Prolonged exposure to noise.
- Family history (think of relatives using hearing aids at a young age, otosclerosis, etc.).
- Previous history: meningitis, ear infections.

Handout is shown on the screen and read aloud.

Stage 2: Results of History Taking
During history taking, Mrs. Mohammed says she doesn't know exactly since when her hearing became worse. It seems that the hearing slowly deteriorated. There is no recent trauma. She was not exposed to noise. She noticed that she often turns up the volume of the television. When she speaks in her native language, the hearing loss does not disappear, but is less evident. As a child she frequently suffered from ear infections. There is no dizziness, but she suffers from tinnitus since several months. She observed no left-right difference.

Question 4   What diagnoses are more likely now?

Hints for Peer Teachers

Insert the data from the handout in the table. Which diagnoses are likely now?

Appendix

Background Information for the Consultant

Here too, a systematic approach is important. Students should think about all the information they have obtained. This information is helpful for making a diagnosis.
See the completed table under the headline *History: pro/against*.
Currently, a disease in the inner ear is most likely.

Question 5 **Which components of the physical examination should you perform? How can these examinations help to distinguish between different diseases?**

Hints for Peer Teachers

Let the students mention what components of physical examination they want to perform. Ask them what findings can be seen related to the different diseases in the differential diagnosis. You should also discuss the tuning fork tests of Rinne and Weber. What is the value of these tests during physical examination? Imagine what a general practitioner (GP) would do.

Background Information for the Consultant

The purpose of the physical examination is to assess the severity and possible causes of the hearing loss. The GP should inspect both ears using an otoscope and pay attention to the following aspects:

- Presence of a cerumen plug or otorrhea in the auditory canal
- Swelling, flaking, redness, vesicles, or erosions of the auditory canal
- Color, opacity, light reflection, and possible perforation of the tympanic membrane
- Presence of a liquid level or air bubble(s) behind the tympanic membrane

Ask them what findings can be seen regarding the different diseases in the differential diagnosis.
In addition, the GP can perform the tuning fork tests of Rinne and Weber. Both experiments and their added value should be discussed.
Using these tests, the origin of the hearing loss can be determined. The sensitivity for the detection of conductive hearing loss is low (both 43 %); the specificity is better (76 % for the test of Weber, 98 % for the test of Rinne). This means that a negative outcome of the test of Rinne (consistent with conductive hearing loss) and a positive Weber to one of the two ears have an additional value to history and physical examination.
Weber: A vibrating tuning fork is put on the middle of the head on the skull. If the patient hears the sound at best at the side of his worst ear, then this could indicate conduction loss in that ear. If the patient hears the sound at best at the side of his better ear, then this indicates having a perception hearing loss of his worst ear.

Rinne: This trial compares the hearing of the tuning fork sound when holding the fork in front of the ear or against the mastoid bone. The outcome is "positive" when the tuning fork is heard better when held in front of the ear (sensorineural deafness or normal hearing). Air conduction is physiologically better than bone conduction. "Negative Rinne" is found when mastoid sound is louder than the sound in front of the ear the ear (pointing at conductive hearing loss).

Handout is shown on the screen and read.

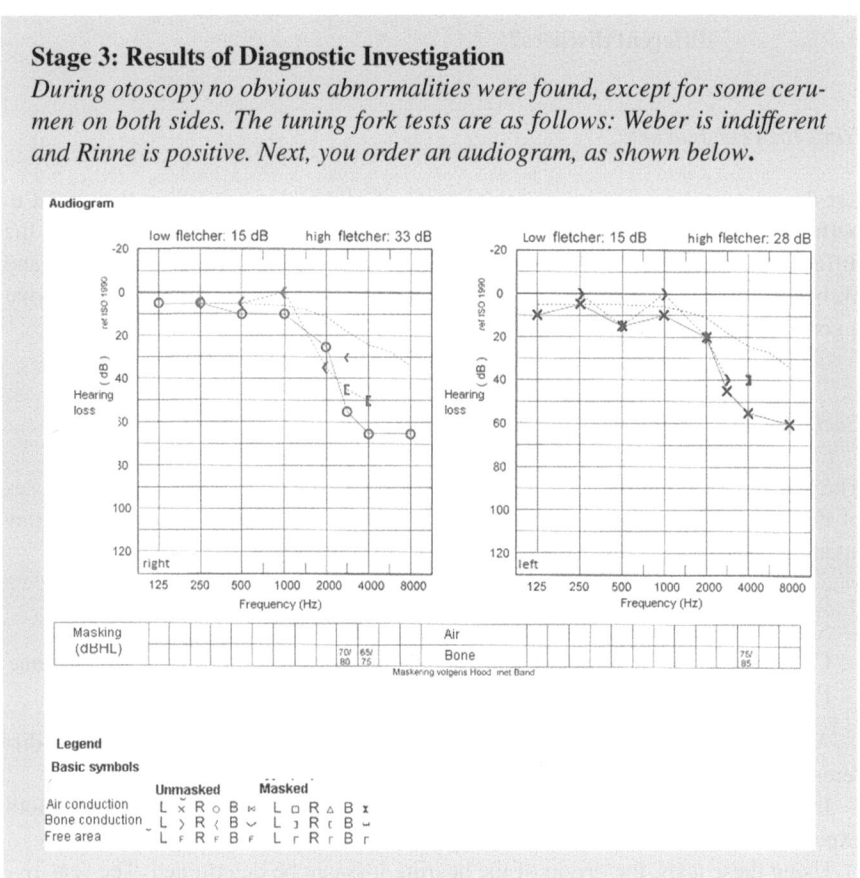

Stage 3: Results of Diagnostic Investigation
During otoscopy no obvious abnormalities were found, except for some cerumen on both sides. The tuning fork tests are as follows: Weber is indifferent and Rinne is positive. Next, you order an audiogram, as shown below.

Question 6   What do the results of the physical examination say? Describe what you see on the audiogram. What is your diagnosis now?

Hints for Peer Teachers

Briefly discuss the findings of physical examination and incorporate these data in the table. What diagnoses will now become more or less likely? Then discuss the findings of the audiogram. Which diagnosis is now most likely?

Appendix 195

Background Information for the Consultant

Otoscopy doesn't show many abnormalities. A little cerumen is definitely not enough for bilateral hearing loss. The tuning fork tests show that air conduction is unaffected (Rinne), so there is normal hearing or sensorineural hearing loss! Weber doesn't lateralize, which tells us hearing of both sides is good or that there is bilateral perception loss.

The audiogram of the handout is a typical example of presbyacusis. Presbyacusis manifests mainly by showing bilateral hearing loss at higher frequencies.

Presbyacusis is a form of sensorineural hearing loss (the condition is therefore in the perception area: cochlea, n. cochlearis, central auditory system). With a sensorineural hearing loss, the conduction loss is equal to the loss of perception. Initially, hearing problems occur mainly at high-frequency sounds; later the hearing of all frequencies is affected.

Question 7   What is your policy with this patient?

Hints for Peer Teachers

What is the best treatment for the diagnosis found in this patient?

Background Information for the Consultant

Information:
   Inform the patient and her environment about:

- Articulating well and speaking in a pace way. Keeping eye contact is a better way to improve communication than increasing speaking volume.
- Acoustics of a room can be improved by the application of absorbent material (carpet on the floor).
- Enhanced telephones or doorbells and tools for TV and radio will reduce the limitations of the patient.

Hearing aid improves the perception of sound, but most hearing aids have trouble distinguishing sound from background noise, so both (signal and noise) will be amplified. Ask for the patient's motivation for a hearing aid. If the patient wants to qualify for a hearing aid, a referral to an otolaryngologist is indicated.

After question 7, one of the peer teachers gives a **mini lecture**.

During the oral presentation, discuss the following causes of hearing loss:

- Unilateral hearing loss (acoustic neuroma or sudden deafness)
- Ototoxicity
- Otosclerosis
- Chronic otitis media with or without cholesteatoma
- Presbyacusis

Discuss in a few words the clinical aspects and specifics of the diseases. What do you find during physical examination (inspection, palpation, tuning fork test, otoscopy)? What is the treatment?

Make sure your lecture lasts no more than 10 min.

	Unilateral hearing loss	Ototoxicity	Otosclerosis	Chronic otitis media with or without cholesteatoma	Presbyacusis
Inspection	No visible anomalies	No visible anomalies	No visible anomalies	Moisture auditory canal	No visible anomalies
Palpation	No anomalies	No anomalies	No anomalies	Pressure pain behind the ear	No anomalies
Assessment of auditory functioning by using tuning fork tests and audiometry screening	Reduced, unilateral	Reduced, mostly bilateral. Weber neutral. Rinne positive	Reduced, mostly unilateral. Weber lateralizes to most affected ear. Rinne negative	Reduced, mostly unilateral. Weber lateralizes to most affected ear. Rinne negative	Reduced, symmetric hearing loss (bilateral)
	Weber lateralizes to healthy ear. Rinne positive				Weber neutral. Rinne positive
Otoscopy	No anomalies	No anomalies	No anomalies	Red tympanic membrane, pus (*not always!*) with perforation (*not always!*)	No anomalies
				Cholesteatoma can be viewed behind the tympanic membrane (accumulation of epidermal skin rests and other epidermal products)	
Treatment	1. Wait and see	Immediately lower the dose of ototoxic medication; preferably prescribe other medication	Surgery: stapedotomy	Chronic otitis media: cleaning of auditory canal and mid ear and application of medication	Hearing aid
	2. Surgery			Cholesteatoma: surgery!	
	3. Stereotactic radiation therapy				

Question 8 **One of the students from the group summarizes the whole case chronologically in a few minutes**

Hints for Peer Teachers

If necessary, you can help the students to summarize using the following format:

During the office hour I saw a … year old man/woman with complaints of … Patient has … as relevant prehistory. Relevant medication is…..

The major problem during history taking is … During the physical examination I saw ….. Additional test showed … (special findings or negative findings). In conclusion, I saw a … year old man/woman with probably … (working diagnosis) for which I want to start … (additional testing or policy). In the differential diagnosis I still consider…..

Background Information for the Consultant

Illness	History		Physical examination		Additional investigations	
	Pro	Against	Pro	Against	Pro	Against
External ear/auditory canal:		No left-right difference				
Cerumen plug				No cerumen plug found by otoscopy		
Otitis externa		No abnormalities of the auditory canal, like otorrhea and (heavy) pain		No conduction loss. (positive test of Rinne)		
Middle ear	Suffering from the ears during childhood	No left-right difference		No abnormalities during otoscopy, test of Weber is indifferent		
Otitis media acuta (OMA)		No fever → can be seen with OMA/COM				
Otitis media with effusion (OME)		No otalgia → can be seen with OMA/COM No otorrhea→ can be seen with COM				
Acute dysfunction van the Eustachian tube		No trauma				
Otitis media chronica=COM (with/without cholesteatoma)						
Myringitis						
Otosclerosis						
Trauma capitis (e.g., tympanic membrane)						

Appendix

Inner ear/cochlear				
Meniere's disease	Tinnitus	No vertigo	No abnormalities during otoscopy, positive test of Rinne, Weber indifferent	
Presbyacusis	Gradual decline of hearing	No ototoxic medications		Audiogram is typical for presbyacusis
Ototoxicity	Disturbed understanding of speech	No exposure to extreme noise		
Noise damage		No trauma		
Trauma capitis (cochlear)				
Retro-cochlear				
Acoustic neuroma	Tinnitus	Bilateral hearing loss		
Trauma capitis (nerve)	Gradual decline of hearing	No trauma		

Case B: A 3-Year-Old Girl With Hearing Loss

Stage 1: Presentation of the Patient's Problem
At your GP office, Mrs. Jones appears with her daughter Sara. Sara is 3 years and 2 months old. You have seen Sara once, 1 year ago, with an ear infection. At the time, you decided to wait and see. Mrs. Jones noticed that Sara hears less since 1 week; she constantly turns the volume of the TV very loud. Also, she was a bit irritable the last few days. Mrs. Jones didn't measure her temperature yet. She once saw Sara grabbing her right ear.

Question 9 Which diagnoses are you considering now? What questions do you need to ask Mrs. Jones?

Hints for Peer Teachers

Use the previously created table.

Background Information for the Consultant

In young children, hearing loss is predominantly caused by otitis media with effusion.

Emphasize that the presentation of these very young children may be nonspecific. The students need to think in large diagnostic groups as in the previously created table. The differential diagnosis of a child with hearing loss (whose further development is normal) reads as follows:

- Otitis media with effusion
- Otitis media acuta
- Cerumen plug
- Otitis externa
- Inner ear pathology or retro-cochlear pathology

  Use the previously created table to formulate the right questions:
  There can still be asked about:

- Moisture from the ear and ear pain (a girl of 3 years old may answer that question herself)
- History of an upper respiratory infection
- Early symptoms of hearing loss and test results from a hear screening test
- Snoring, reduced nasal patency, and open-mouth breathing (because of large adenoid)
- Nursery/day care

Appendix

- Other children in family
- Other symptoms such as asthma, bronchitis, eczema, and allergies
- Severity, duration, and course of symptoms
- Speech and language development
- Trauma?

Question 10 Do you want to perform a physical examination? If so, what would you examine?

Hints for Peer Teachers

What kind of physical examination do you want to perform? How do you judge the auditory canal and tympanic membrane? What would you pay attention to?

Background Information for the Consultant

During physical examination it is especially important to judge the general impression of the child. Does she look sick and/or painful? Is she cranky or can she still laugh? It is also important to get an impression of the ENT (ear-nose-throat) area by inspection of the ear, the auditory canal, and tympanic membrane using an otoscope.

Attention should be paid to swelling, flaking, redness, otorrhea, vesicles, and erosions of the external auditory canal. The tympanic membrane should be judged on color (pink, bright, or dull), position (withdrawn, normal, bulging), transparency, light reflection, and any (rare) presence of a liquid surface or air bubble(s).

In addition, look for other possible signs of infection: fever, swollen glands, stuffy nose, etc.

Also, the doctor should look for signs that may indicate complications: surrendered position of the ear, a painful mastoid during pressure, stiff neck, or impaired consciousness.

Handout is now displayed on the screen and read out loud.

Stage 2: Results of History Taking and Physical Examination
Sara indeed complains about ear pain and points at her right ear. She has a bad cold since a few days. Mrs. Jones did not see any moisture running from the ear, as she saw with the pervious episode. Her speech and language development don't cause any concerns.

Using the otoscope you see a red, bulging tympanic membrane, at the right as well the left side, but right> left. The tuning fork tests show the following: Rinne is negative on the right; Weber lateralizes to the right. Her temperature is 38.2 °C.

Question 11   What is your diagnosis and what will be your policy?

Hints for Peer Teachers

What is for now the most likely diagnosis?

What will be the treatment? Do not only think of drug therapy but also relate to the underlying pathology (adenoid, tonsils).

The six-step model is a tool that allows you to determine the treatment systematically in six steps from diagnosis. Let your colleague students practice in writing a recipe.

Background Information for the Consultant

Acute otitis media is most likely. The tuning fork test shows conduction loss, which matches this diagnosis. A completed six-step plan can be found in the appendices. The students and peer teachers will receive a noncompleted version of the case. Important is the rational choice of a medicament for this patient. A recipe contains at least the name of the patient; date; including the drug dose; number of prescribed tablets; prescription; and a signature.

NB. In case of recurrent otitis: Consider hypertrophy of the adenoid and tonsils. Conservative treatment consists of cleaning the nose with saline or a short-term treatment with xylometazoline nose spray (0.05 % for children <6 years). An adenoidectomy should be considered when there are persistent infective/obstructive symptoms of adenoid and/or middle ear problems, which affect the general health and child development adversely.

Question 11:   One of the students from the group summarizes the whole case chronologically in a few minutes

Hints for Peer Teachers

If necessary, you can help the students to summarize using the following format:

During the office hour I saw a … year old man/woman with complaints of … Patient has … as relevant prehistory. Relevant medication is…..

The major problem during history taking is … During the physical examination I saw ….. Additional test showed … (special findings or negative findings). In conclusion, I saw a … year old man/woman with probably … (working diagnosis) for which I want to start … (additional testing or policy). In the differential diagnosis I still consider…..

Appendix

Background Information for the Consultant

Illness	History		Physical examination		Additional investigations	
	Pro	Against	Pro	Against	Pro	Against
External ear/ auditory canal	Otalgia→ external otitis	No otorrhea→ otitis externa		Auditory canal is not closed by cerumen		
Cerumen plug						
Otitis externa						
Middle ear:	Lethargic, fever, recent inflammations Otalgia	No trauma	Fever, lethargic, very red bulging tympanic membrane			
Otitis media acuta (OMA)	Upper respiratory infection since a couple of days		Rinne negative right ear, Weber lateralizes to the right			
Otitis media with effusion (OME)						
Acute dysfunction van the Eustachian tube						
Otitis media chronica = COM (with/ without cholesteatoma)						
Myringitis						
Otosclerosis						
Trauma capitis (e.g., tympanic membrane)						
Inner ear/ cochlear		Too young, no noise damage, no trauma		Negative test of Rinne		
Meniere's disease						
Presbyacusis						
Ototoxicity						
Noise damage trauma capitis (cochlear)						
Retro-cochlear		Too young, no trauma		Negative test of Rinne		
Acoustic neuroma						
Trauma capitis (nerve)						

Index

A
Abduction, 37
Abstraction, 37, 38, 49, 53
Advanced teaching certificate, 115
Analytical thinking, 4, 5
Anchoring bias, 6, 43
Aphorisms, 22
Arrangement, 14, 76
Artificial intelligence (AI), 26, 36
Availability bias, 6, 43

B
Backward-driven reasoning, 38
Batista de Monte, 22
Bayesian probability, 8
Beside teaching, 22
Blackboard, 61, 76, 102
Boerhaave, H., 22
Bond, T., 23
Bounded rationality bias, 43
Branched programming, 25, 26

C
Case-based clinical reasoning in practice, 75–82
Case-based clinical reasoning test, 67
Case-based collaborative learning, 15
Case-based discussion (CBD), 67
Case selection, 58
Case specificity, 26, 27, 41, 86
CBCR consultants, 96, 114
CBCR peer teachers, 77, 79
CBCR session, 12, 75, 77–79, 81, 82, 86, 88, 96, 116, 117, 123
CBCR session participation points, 130–131
CBCR study guide, 81
Central processing unit, 36
Chart-stimulated recall (CSR), 67
Chronology of the present illness, 51
Chunks, 12, 38, 39
Clinical decision support systems (CDSS), 36
Clinical problem analysis (CPA), 29
Clinical reasoning, v, 3, 21, 23–30, 35–44, 47–54, 57–61, 66–70, 85–89, 91, 109–118, 122–132
Clinical reasoning problems' test, 67
Clinical vocabulary, 14, 48–51, 53, 54, 61
Cognitive biases, 7
Cognitive load, 12, 13, 30
Comprehensive integrative puzzle test, 67
Computer-assisted instruction (CAI), 25, 26
Confirmation bias, 43
Consequences, 3, 5, 12, 13, 27, 37, 39, 42, 54, 57, 59, 60, 66, 163
Consultant version, 11, 77, 81, 97
Consultant version of the CBCR case, 11, 97
Contrastive learning, 14, 48, 58
Course conditions, 75–77
Course development, 112–114
Course directors, 80–82, 111, 114
Credit points, 121, 122
Curriculum description, 110
Curriculum development, 10, 109–112
Curriculum framework, 110, 111
Curriculum governance, 111
Curriculum planning, 76

D

Deduction, 37, 38
Deliberate practice, 9, 42
Delivered curriculum, 110
Diagnostic drill, 26
Diagnostic errors, 7, 43
Diagnostic problem solving, 4, 24, 28
Diagnostic verification, 6, 14, 48, 60–62
Differential diagnosis, vi, 7, 23, 28–30, 37, 43, 54, 58, 66, 69, 85, 87, 89, 98, 102, 103, 117, 123, 124, 126, 142, 147
Discriminating information, 48
Disease manifestation matrix, 25
Dual process theory, 4, 40

E

Electronic testing, 67
Empirium, 29
Enabling conditions, 5, 12, 13, 57, 59
Encapsulation of knowledge, 40
Experienced curriculum, 110
Extended matching questions' test, 67
Extraneous load, 30
The eyeball test, 36

F

Facet, 29
Facilities, 76, 110, 111, 114
Faculty development, 81, 109–118
Fault, 5, 6, 12, 39, 57, 59
Flexner, A., 8, 23–25
Flip chart, 102
Forward-driven reasoning, 38

G

Galen, 22
Germane load, 30
Global complex, 29
Group dynamics, 77, 81
Guidelines for effective case writing, 95
GUIDON-MANAGE, 27

H

Handouts, 11, 76, 77, 102, 103, 106, 126
Heuristics, 4, 22, 43
Hidden curriculum, 110
Hippocratean-Galenic medical theory, 21–23
Hippocrates, 22
Humoral theory, 22
Hypothesis-driven inquiry, 14, 48, 54, 59–61
Hypothesis generation, 28, 38, 52

I

Illness script, 4, 5, 8, 9, 12–14, 38, 39, 54, 57, 59–61, 65, 69, 83, 86, 96, 98
Illness script mental repository, 14, 48, 54–58, 61, 66
Induction, 28, 37, 38
Instances, vi, 38, 39, 41, 50, 53, 76
Intelligent tutoring systems (ITS), 26
Intermediate effect, 40
Internists, 27, 36, 41
Intuition, 36

J

Judging by similarity, 43

K

Kern's six-step approach to currriculum development, 110, 112

L

Learner domain space, 36
Leyden University, 22
Logoscope, 25
Long menu questions, 68, 69, 88
Long-term memory, 5, 12, 13, 38–40, 52, 54, 58, 60–62, 86

M

Management, 4, 5, 7, 9, 12, 13, 48, 54, 69, 80–82, 86, 97, 98, 110, 145, 163
Medical decision-making, 8
Medical problem solving, 25, 28, 29, 37, 41
Miller's pyramid, 111
Mini clinical evaluation exercise, 67
Mini-lectures, 78, 97, 104, 127, 128, 145, 160
Mission statement, 110, 111
Modernizing Undergraduate Medical Education in the Eastern Neighboring Area (MUMEENA), v, 115
MYCIN, 27, 36

N

Near-peer consultants, 82
Neuroscience, 43
Nonanalytic reasoning, 65

O

Obduction, 23
Objectives, 4, 30, 65, 67, 77, 82, 85, 95, 97, 109–113, 122, 123
Objective structured clinical examination (OSCE), 66
Osler, W., 23, 24, 30
Outcome bias, 43

P

Participant roles, 76, 78–80
Patient assessment and management examination (PAME), 67
Patient management problem (PMP), 25, 26, 69
Patient-oriented thinking, 10–12
Pattern recognition, 4, 9, 12, 28, 40, 65, 66
Peer teacher version, v, 77, 79, 80, 96, 97, 124, 126, 129
Peer teacher version of the CBCR case, 11
Peer teaching, v, 14, 160
PhD diploma in health professions education research, 115
Planned curriculum, 110
Postgraduate scholarly educator certificate, 115
Pre-Hippocratic era, 21
Premature closure, 6, 29, 43
Problem-based learning (PBL), 4, 15, 26, 27, 48, 80, 95
Problem-oriented medical record, 29
Problem representation, 7, 14, 48, 52–59, 61, 62, 69
Progress test, 65
Projection screens, 76
Prototypes, 13, 38, 39, 175
Prototype theory, 38
Pseudodiagnosticity, 43

Q

Quality assurance, 80, 110–112

R

Reasoning, 3, 21, 23–30, 35–44, 47–54, 57–61, 66–70, 85–89, 91, 109–118, 122–132
Reflection in action, 42
Reflection on action, 42

Reliability, 68–70, 87
Representative bias, 43
Response process, 66
Retrospective bias, 30
Roadmap to clinical decision-making, 124
Rooms, 76
Rules for repeaters, 132
Rules for the exam retake, 132

S

Scenarios, 86, 87, 89, 107, 118
Scheduling groups, 75–76
Schemas, 38, 58, 62
Scientific discovery, 36
Script activation, 39
Script concordance testing, 67, 68, 86, 88
Scripts, 5, 39
Search satisficing, 43
Semantically driven discourse, 50
Semantic networks, 38
Semantic qualifiers, 7, 38, 39, 49–54, 61, 69
Short-answer open questions' test, 67
Situated cognition, 41
Situated learning, 41
Situativity, 41
SPICES, 112
Standardized oral examination, 67
Standardized patient station, 67
Structured reflection, 42
Student instruction, 118
Student teaching certificate, 115
Student version, 77, 96, 97, 124
Student version of CBCR case, 11
Symptom-driven discourse, 60
System 1 and 2 thinking, 4, 40
System-oriented thinking, 11–12

T

Teacher training course, 82
Teaching certificates, 115
Team-based learning (TBL), 15
Template for CBCR Cases, 99

V

Validity of educational and psychological tests, 66

W

Working memory, 12
Written case summaries, 67, 69

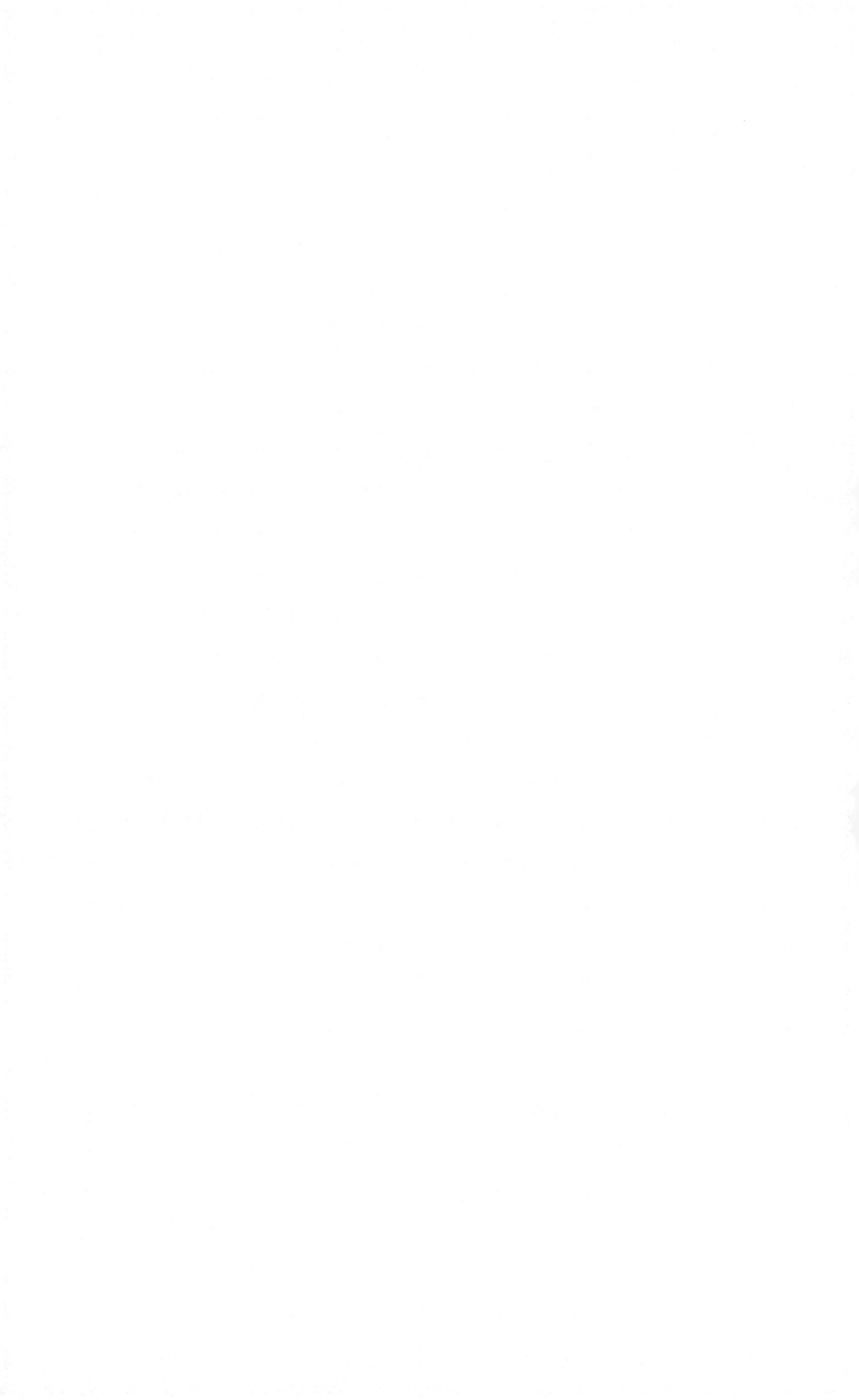

The manufacturer's authorised representative in the EU is Springer Nature Customer Service Centre GmbH, Europaplatz 3, 69115 Heidelberg, Germany. If you have any concerns regarding our products, please contact ProductSafety@springernature.com

Printed and bound by CPI Group (UK) Ltd, Croydon, CR0 4YY

26/03/2026

02078975-0001